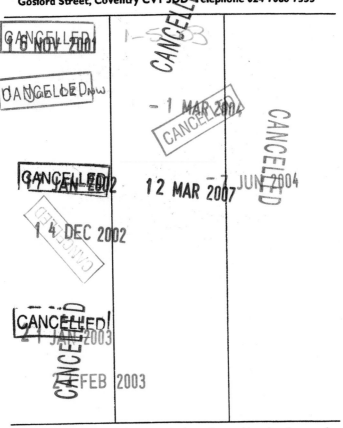
This book is due to be returned not later than the date and
time stamped above. Fines are charged on overdue books

Handbook of Mobilization in the Management of Children with Neurologic Disorders

Handbook of Mobilization in the Management of Children with Neurologic Disorders

Sandra Brooks-Scott, Ed.D., PPT, PCS

President, Pediatric Physical Therapy, Inc.,
Hazelwood, Missouri

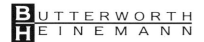

Boston   Oxford   Auckland   Johannesburg   Melbourne   New Delhi

GLOBAL   Butterworth–Heinemann supports the efforts of American Forests and the
RELEAF   Global ReLeaf program in its campaign for the betterment of trees, forests, and
2000   our environment.

Library of Congress Cataloging-in-Publication Data
Brooks-Scott, Sandra.
    Handbook of mobilization in the management of children with
neurologic disorders / Sandra Brooks-Scott.
        p.   cm.
    Includes bibliographical references and index.
    ISBN 0-7506-7025-8
    1. Movement disorders in children--Treatment. 2. Nervous system-
-Diseases--Physical therapy. 3. Physical therapy for children.
4. Occupational therapy for children. I. Title.
    [DNLM: 1. Nervous System Diseases--in infancy & childhood.
2. Nervous System Diseases--complications. 3. Motor Skills
Disorders--in infancy & childhood. 4. Physical Therapy--in infancy
& childhood. 5. Occupational Therapy--in infancy & childhood. WS
340 B873h 1999]
RJ496.M68B76 1999
618.92'8--dc21
DNLM/DLC
for Library of Congress   98-32457
                                                              CIP

British Library Cataloguing-in-Publication Data
A catalogue record for this book is available from the British Library.

The publisher offers special discounts on bulk orders of this book.

For information, please contact: For information on all Butterworth–Heinemann
Manager of Special Sales   publications available, contact our World Wide Web
Butterworth–Heinemann   home page at: http://www.bh.com
225 Wildwood Avenue
Woburn, MA 01801-2041
Tel: 781-904-2500
Fax: 781-904-2620

10 9 8 7 6 5 4 3 2 1

Printed in the United States of America

To Ryan

Contents

Preface

Designed to be both clinically relevant and practical, this book was written for therapists trying to balance the myriad of theories with the demands of real life in their treatment of young patients. It examines the history of therapy for children with neurologic disorders and the evolution of commonly used theoretic approaches; it also discusses current motor theory, combining orthopedic and neurologic perspectives to make feasible the goal of efficient movement. It puts a traditional approach in a new light, raising issues to be addressed based on a child's specific circumstances, not on diagnosis. Finally, the text addresses controversial issues (e.g., the knowledge that therapy cannot go on forever and that therapy may not be the best or most efficient means to achieve a motor skill) that therapists address every day. I hope this text helps therapists illuminate the issues, formulate the questions, gather the data, and analyze the results needed to provide cost-effective, efficient interventions that enable their patients to move as efficiently as possible without detracting from other aspects of quality living.

In 1983, I was taking an advanced course in a popular neurologic approach. That approach was used to treat a boy with severe quadriplegia from cerebral palsy. His progress at that point had been minimal, and the orthopedic surgery scheduled for him was considered his only opportunity to improve. Mobilization was performed as an adjunct to the neurologic approach, because it could not hurt the child and might provide some mobility. The boy experienced significant improvement in motor abilities and did not need as invasive a surgery. Theoretically, an orthopedic technique would have no effect on the child's motor behavior. It did, however, thus beginning the search for alternative explanations of limited motor behavior and treatments of motor impairment subsequent to neurologic damage.

Traditional neurologic approaches focus on the contribution of the nervous system to movement and its disorders. By presenting movement disorders from a systems, not solely a diagnostic, perspective, this text suggests alternative causes of motor impairment in children with neurologic disorders; these alternatives must be considered to effectively treat a patient's movement pattern. This book is not about the treatment of cerebral palsy, spina bifida, or spinal muscular atrophy; rather, it is about proximate causes and treatment methods for the motor dysfunction that such disorders cause.

The text is organized to flow from the academic perspective of traditional neurologic approaches (Chapter 1) through current neurologic theory (Chapter 2). Because current neurologic theory acknowledges the role of neurology and biomechanics, Chapters 3 and 4 review principles of biomechanics and orthopedics for the neurologically oriented therapist. The academic perspective is put into clinical terms in Chapters 5 and 6, as theories are directly applied to the assessment and treatment planning for seven case examples. Finally, in Chapter 7, the clinical perspective is tailored to the business perspective of medical efficiency and fiscal responsibility. The student will readily relate to the first four chapters; the new graduate will relate to the fifth and sixth chapters; the experienced clinician, however, must balance the first six chapters with the realities of the world outside of therapy and will appreciate the issues raised in the seventh chapter.

Each chapter uses the same case examples to illustrate key points. Those case examples are presented in Chapter 6. Although their names have been changed, these are actual children I have treated. Practicing therapists will readily identify with these children and with the complexity of the issues surrounding not just their quality of movement but also their quality of life.

Sandra Brooks-Scott

1

Historical Perspective

Physical and occupational therapy for children with neurologic disabilities has changed dramatically since the early half of the twentieth century. At that time, rehabilitation of children with polio had a distinct orthopedic flavor. Stretching and bracing were the techniques of choice to correct orthopedic deformity resulting from viral damage to the peripheral nervous system. With the widespread use of the polio vaccine, fewer children with polio are seen in therapy clinics. On another front, advancements in prenatal and neonatal medicine have allowed more premature infants to survive. However, many of these prematurely born infants who survived had central nervous system damage. Therapeutic intervention for the sequelae of this damage grew from the foundation of management of polio and in the orthopedic concepts of stretching and bracing.

With the shift from peripheral nervous system damage to central nervous system damage, changes in theories of motor control shifted the emphasis of therapy from orthopedic management of deformity subsequent to neurologic damage to neurologic strategies to improve motor control. Key theorists providing therapeutic approaches based on motor control theories were Bobath (1980) and the neurodevelopmental treatment (NDT) approach, Stockmeyer (1967) and the sensorimotor approach, and Voss (1985) with the proprioceptive neuromuscular facilitation (PNF). A more recent therapeutic approach based on later neurologic studies was developed by Ayres (1972) in the sensory integration model.

These approaches provide the background to address current variations of therapy presented in this text. As such, each approach and its underlying neurologic constructs are briefly reviewed. Chapter 2 discusses a different perspective of motor control; subsequent chapters suggest additional approaches to therapeutic management of children with neurologic disorders.

NDT, the sensorimotor approach, and PNF are different treatment regimens built on similar neurologic principles. NDT became more popular for those treating infants as it relied more on "handling" and automatic movements. The sensorimotor approach was readily adapted for both children and adults, whereas PNF had specific movement patterns that were difficult to use with infants and small children. At the time these approaches were developed, motor control theory focused on reflexive or primitive vs. voluntary or coordinated movement. Brain damage interfered with the primitive postural control that formed the base for mature voluntary movement. Because the brain recognized movement, not muscles (John Hughlings in Jackson and Taylor 1932), normal patterns of movement such as automatic reactions provided the foundation on which voluntary and purposeful movement could be facilitated. Habits of normal movement replaced the abnormal movement of the child with brain damage, thereby "preventing an increase in spasticity or athetosis" (Pearson and Williams 1972, p. 44).

Normal motor development was discussed in terms of the "gradual appearance of the normal postural reflex mechanism and the elaboration and modification of the early primitive total synergies of movement" (Pearson and Williams 1972, p. 44). Pearson and Williams go on:

> *Essentially, normal child development is characterized by two features which are as follows:*
>
> *1. The development in a definite sequence of events of a normal postural reflex mechanism (that is, of righting), equilibrium and other protective reactions, associated with a normal postural tone.*

2. The increase of inhibition of the maturing brain leading to a gradual breaking up and resynthesis of the early total synergies of muscular coordination in many and varied ways to allow for discreet and selective movements later on (p. 44).

Traditional theories of motor control suggest a hierarchic framework in which stereotypic or reflexive movements provide a base of movement patterns early in development on which higher level voluntary movement is built. According to Sherrington's (1906) work, reflexes and reactions formed the building blocks of voluntary movement patterns. Normal motor development was conceived as "a highly automated and consistent progression within the species from rolling to sitting, crawling, standing and walking" (Keshner 1991, p. 39). Therefore, damage to the central nervous system was understood to release lower or more primitive motor patterns. Treatment approaches for children as well as for adults with acquired central nervous system damage often focused on repeating the normal developmental sequence. As Keshner points out, "[t]he weakness in this belief is that it reflects a primacy of neural structure over function and fails to acknowledge the consistencies inherent in other aspects of development" (p. 39). The relationship between function and adapting structure was posited by Piaget and Inhelder (1969) and documented in studies of environmental enrichment as well as sensory deprivation. The automatic and consistent progression of motor skills does not reflect the individual variation in timing of motor skills (as seen in tests of motor development such as the Bailey Scales of Infant Development and the Denver Developmental Screening Test) and variability in order of appearance of motor skills (Bottos et al. 1989; Robson 1984) within a culture nor the intercultural variations documented in the literature (Malina 1998; Super 1976; Thorton 1992).

From this perspective, a focus on reflexes, reactions, facilitation, and inhibition pervaded therapy. Because normal development was conceptualized as a fixed pattern of motor skills emerging at predetermined times as the brain matured, and brain damage interfered with this predetermined pattern, therapy focused on inhibiting abnormal tone, facilitating normal righting and balance reactions, and moving the child (and adult) through the normal developmental sequence of motor skills. Gone were orthopedic principles of bracing and muscle stretching. Therapy was often viewed as a failure when orthopedic approaches including surgery were necessary.

Although NDT and PNF were grounded in similar neurologic theory, they developed very different treatment techniques to address the motor problems. NDT focused on the nervous system and its theoretical primitive reflexes and equilibrium reactions as a base for techniques to develop normal posture and movement, whereas PNF techniques were more focused on the triplanar nature of muscles and their actions. By placing joints and limbs in specific positions, muscle action could be facilitated or inhibited by applying resistance or assistance to synergistic muscle groups. An extensive array of diagonal movement patterns were identified and formed the basis of the PNF techniques. The bias of each theory's focus produced different treatment techniques.

Shifts in focus produced additional treatment techniques from Margaret Rood as documented by Stockmeyer (1967). Shirley Stockmeyer documented the slightly different focus taken by Rood in the sensorimotor approach to treatment. The focus in this approach addressed the interrelationships among motor, cognitive, and affective domains. Development was seen as moving from a protective avoidance stage to a stage of interacting with the environment. Two systems were posited: One system included the sensorimotor mechanisms that allow movement free of weightbearing, whereas the other system included sensorimotor mechanisms affecting posture in weightbearing. This first mechanism was described as phasic or dynamic; the second was conceived of as tonic or postural. The treatment modalities of this approach focused more on types of sensory stimuli and the child's reaction to that stimuli. Once the correct reaction was obtained, it was built on with a progression of nonweightbearing, then weightbearing, activities to produce voluntary motor control.

A. Jean Ayres (1972) extended this focus on the role of sensory input to produce normal motor output in her theory of sensory integration. Her treatment techniques were based on the inter-relationships among different sensory systems to produce normal motion. Hence, vestibular, tactile, and proprioceptive information are all processed to allow adaptive motor responses to environmental stimuli. Imbalance in these systems produces maladaptive motor and emotional behavior. Techniques attributed to this approach focus on eliciting normal responses to both individual sensory input and combinations thereof.

All of these perspectives have a few points in common. First, the brain directs the movement based on sensory input. Second, patterns of responses built into the brain are released in pre-dictable time frames and form the basis of normal movement. Finally, the focus is on the brain. The rest of the body systems sim-ply respond to the normal or abnormal behavior directed by the brain. As is discussed in subsequent chapters, these tenets have been called into question. Note that, although the tenets have been called into question, this in no way invalidates the techniques.

Fay Horak (1991) clearly states the dilemma faced by thera-pists. These theoretical perspectives are based on assumptions about motor control. "These assumptions shape, structure, and limit therapist's observations and treatments of their neurologi-cally impaired patients" (p. 11). Alternative theories of motor con-trol provide the opportunity to reshape, restructure, and expand the limits of the therapist's observations and treatments. In that light, Chapter 2 addresses current theories of motor control.

2

Theories of Motor Control

Chapter 1 addressed traditional theories of motor control and their influence on theories of therapeutic intervention. This chapter presents theories of motor control including feedback and feed-forward systems, motor programs, and systems of motor control.

Feedback and Feed-Forward Systems

The discussion of motor control in Chapter 1 was based on four assumptions that, with the advance of research techniques, have been called into question.

1. Reflexes are the building blocks of movement.

2. Sensory feedback is required for movement.

3. Skills develop in a fixed and predictable sequence.

4. Motor control develops in a cephalocaudal direction.

Considerable evidence suggests these assumptions are too simplistic.

Reflexes, the tightly coupled sensory input–motor output circuits, are the basis of many therapeutic techniques. Reflex pathways are necessary circuits in the nervous system; the pathways can be reorganized for many types of movement. Although reflexes and voluntary movement share some of the same neural pathways, evidence shows that coordinated movement is not controlled by reflexes (Bradley and Bekoff 1989; Towen 1984).

The second assumption—that sensory feedback is required for movement—has also been questioned. Both feedback and feed-forward systems produce movement. Feedback of sensory information is necessary for motor learning (Schmidt 1991) and to adjust to changing environmental demands (Polit and Bizzi 1979). Once a skill is learned, motor control is executed with feed-forward loops (Schmidt 1991). Guiliani (1991) states that "[a]lthough the sensory information is available during rapid movements, it cannot be used to perform the movement because the movement proceeds faster than the nervous system can process and use the sensory information" (p. 30). Hence, highly coordinated skills, such as playing the piano, have limited reliance on sensory input.

Motor Programs

The feed-forward, or open loop, concept of motor control is necessary for motor program control. A motor program is a movement sequence with given variant and invariant features that is stored in the nervous system (Schmidt 1991). Walking is a classic example. The sequence and timing of the muscle action are the same for a range of walking speeds, as "coded" in the motor program in the neural circuitry, but speed and direction of the walk can be varied.

Although the nervous system circuitry is important for motor control, Bernstein (1967) notes the additional importance of the contribution of the musculoskeletal system. Changes in limb length (e.g., growth or the addition of a splint on one limb) directly impair motor accuracy. Bernstein posited that the inherent properties of the musculoskeletal system directly influence motor control (Tuller et al. 1982; Turvey et al. 1982). His perspective has generated theories grouped under the term *dynamic systems theory*.

Dynamic Systems

Dynamic systems theory is a term used by many disciplines, with different meanings. Guiliani (1991) describes the theory as the study of complex systems through the *interaction* of subsystems (such as biological, cognitive, social environmental, perceptual, and memory) in the production of behavior. This perspective of motor control is based on Bernstein's observation (1967) that the study of movement must take into account all forces acting on a limb, not just the nervous system. Guiliani (1991) cites the swing phase of gait as an example. During swing phase, very little muscle activity is necessary, yet the movement is well coordinated among all of the joints. Bernstein's perspective suggests this characteristic is due to factors inherent in the limb, such as viscoelastic properties of the muscles and tendons, gravity, momentum, and intersegmental forces. In this example, the nervous system is only a minor contributor to motor control. Bernstein suggested that the multiple degrees of freedom (i.e., each element of the system including muscles, bones, joints, and neural circuitry) are constrained to act as a coordinating structure by the viscoelastic properties of muscle, the composition of tendons and ligaments, the shapes of joints, and other intrinsic structural factors (Tuller et al. 1982; Turvey et al. 1982).

Based on the work of Bernstein (1967), Sporns and Edelman (1993) identified three challenges to previous theories of motor control.

1.   Evolutionary changes in the musculoskeletal system must be accompanied by changes in the nervous system. Because it is unlikely that changes in one system will be accompanied by the spontaneous, but unrelated change in the other system of any given individual, Sporns and Edelman suggest that the nervous system must be able to adapt to peripheral biomechanical changes.

2.   The large variability of motion (i.e., variability beyond the small repertoire of learned movements) is specified redundantly in the nervous system. An example of redundant specification is the ability to write with the right hand, with the left hand, or with a mouth stick.

3.   Coordination is not innate but develops during the postnatal period in response to huge variations in neural and biomechanical, as well as environmental, factors.

Motor coordination is "the process of mastering redundant degrees of freedom of the moving organ," according to Bernstein

(1967, p. 127). Degrees of freedom include each joint and all the directions in which it can move; each muscle and all the actions it can perform; and each neural pathway and all the ways in which it can influence other pathways, muscles, and joints. For a movement to be functional, many other movement possibilities must be limited.

Sporns and Edelman (1993) suggest that the development of motor coordination occurs in response to growth in both the brain and the musculoskeletal systems. Neuronal group selection considers how that coordination occurs. Neuronal groups are circuits of loosely interconnected neurons that share functional properties. These groups may, for example, represent the body surface on the cortex or visual space. Although the groups are distinct, they are also reciprocally interconnected. Selection of these groups can lead to reinforcement or diminution (groups not selected) of responses, allowing categorization of sensory inputs and integration of sensorimotor processes to produce functional behavior.

Sporns and Edelman (1993) suggest that coordination depends on three concurrent variables:

1. Spontaneous generation of a variety of movements

2. Ability to sense the effects of movement, allowing movement selection based on function

3. Selection of functional movement, reinforcing the synaptic connections in the neural circuits

Selection of movement patterns of neuromusculoskeletal units is reinforced if there is an adaptive value (i.e., the motion is functional). These patterns between the neural, muscular, and skeletal systems adapt not only to changes within the systems themselves (e.g., growth) but also to changes in the performance of apparently similar tasks (e.g., picking up an empty vs. a full bottle). These multisystem synergies produce a repertoire of functional movement from which the child can discover, then explore, and ultimately quickly choose to interact with the environment—as opposed to requiring the brain to calculate and control every step of each task. As this basic repertoire of functional neuromusculoskeletal synergies is produced, its use can then be modified for given tasks.

Thelen et al. (1993) support Sporns and Edelman's theory. Thelen et al. propose that infant motion develops in a dynamic and context-specific manner using whatever intrinsic components (e.g., force production or musculoskeletal stiffness) that individual has available. These intrinsic components are specific to the individual—that is, some children have more (or less) ability to produce force and more (or less) musculoskeletal stiffness than other children. Because each child has unique combinations of intrinsic components with which to learn to interact in the environment, the strategies used to harness these unique components must be specific to that child. Thelen et al. (1993) focused on the skill of reaching. They suggest that skill emerges from a discovery and exploration of components available to perform a task. Hence, in reaching, necessary components include visual location of a toy in space, intention to interact with the toy, improved control of the head and trunk, and the "increasing ability to modulate the force and compliance of the arms" (p. 1093).

The order of the appearance of the components (strict developmental sequence) is not critical to success in the skill. In fact, in their longitudinal study of six children, Thelen et al. (1993) reported that each child had an individual approach to discovery of, and adaptation to, the internal characteristics of his or her individual neuromusculoskeletal systems before the skill of reaching occurred. Even after the skill emerged, the children were adjusting their muscular force and arm stiffness to the environmental interaction of the moment. Thelen et al. (1993) suggest that the central nervous system adjusts the dynamic aspects of the limb as opposed to calculating trajectories or muscle firing patterns.

A corollary to this theory is that damage to the brain may alter the brain's ability to adjust intrinsic factors of the limb such as muscle force and joint stiffness. Chapter 3 discusses these intrinsic factors from a biomechanical perspective; Chapter 4 addresses therapeutic approaches to changing the intrinsic factors.

3

Biomechanics of Motor Control

Chapters 1 and 2 have explained that motor control requires coordination among the systems. This coordination includes neural maturation, biomechanical and musculoskeletal development, and the behavioral expression. Chapter 2 focuses on advances in motor control from a neurologic perspective; this chapter advances the discussion of the contribution of biomechanics and musculoskeletal development on motor control.

Some authors have labeled the interaction among the systems producing motor control *biodynamics*, based on the work of Nicholas Bernstein. Bernstein proposed that "motor coordination and control emerged from continual and intimate interactions between the nervous system and the periphery, the limbs and body segments" (Lockman and Thelen 1993, p. 954). In contrast to the traditional theories of motor development in which the brain commands the motor response, Bernstein posited that, for the organism to respond to a changing environment, interaction between the brain and the biomechanical properties of the body must be ongoing. Hence, instead of focusing on prepatterned reflexes or motor programs, the focus shifted to understanding the relationship between the brain and biomechanics of moving limbs. This chapter presents the updated research on understanding the brain-biomechanics interaction. A refresher on biomechanics is followed by the application of these concepts toward the understanding of control of reach in adults. Finally, these principles are applied to development of reach in infancy.

Review of Biomechanics

"Biomechanics is the application of the principles and methods of mechanics to the study of biological systems" (Zernicke and Schneider 1993, p. 982). Biomechanics involves the physics of motion applied to living tissues. Mechanics can be subdivided into kinematics and dynamics. Kinematics focuses on forces of motion, whereas dynamics addresses the physical causes for changes in motion. Kinematic variables such as position, linear and angular velocity, and acceleration can be linked with the electromyographic recordings made during motion. Dynamic variables include force, torque, and power.

Two types of forces exist—external and internal. Examples of external forces include gravity, friction at contact points, and weights. Internal forces include active force from the muscles and passive forces provided by ligaments, periarticular connective tissue, and joints.

Passive Components of the Musculoskeletal System

Bone is composed of compact and cancellous tissue. The dense compact bone and trabecular meshwork of cancellous bone are tissues that can resist tension, compression, and shear forces, usually at the same time. Referring to Wolff's law, bone is a dynamic tissue capable of modeling based on stresses (or lack thereof) placed on it. Weightbearing and muscle contraction are two main forces responsible for modeling bone. Active exercise can increase or decrease bone weight, length, and density, depending on the age of the subject and intensity of the exercise. Lack of exercise from disuse, immobility, weakness, or neurologic damage also affects bone. Bone resorption as opposed to a decrease in bone formation may be responsible for the loss of density seen from disuse (Cornwall, 1984).

The articular cartilage covering the bone has two functions: (1) dissipating the loads applied to the joints and (2) minimizing friction between the opposing surfaces. Because of its composition of 60% water and 40% layered matrix of collagen and proteoglycan gel, articular cartilage can accept high compressive forces. Exercise appears to thicken the cartilage. Repetitive and excessive stress concentrated on small areas can cause tissue failure. Immobility, whether from casting or weakness from neurologic insult, produces tissue changes such as ulcerations and matrix fibrillations. These changes produce abnormal loading, friction, and pressure.

Collagenous tissues include ligaments and periarticular connective tissue, tendons, and skin. Collagenous tissue absorbs tensile forces. The more parallel the fibers, the more tensile force the tissue can absorb. Hence, tendons absorb the most force, whereas skin absorbs the least. To absorb the stress and limit motion in a particular direction, ligaments frequently form from thickenings of the periarticular connective tissue in which the collagen fibers are arranged in a more parallel fashion than other parts of the tissue. The amount and size of collagen fibers increase with exercise and decrease with immobility (Cornwall 1984). Deformities in children with cerebral palsy may be the result of abnormal stresses from incorrect joint alignment (Bleck 1982; Cusick 1990).

Muscle tissue also responds to stress. The fiber properties and compliance of tissue is influenced by activity, or lack thereof. Tardieu and Tardieu (1987) showed that tissues lost sarcomeres after immobilization of the muscle. The resulting decrease in muscle compliance (i.e., stiffness) was not due to neural damage but to muscle tissue changes. In this example, increased resistance to passive stretch would have had nothing to do with a disruption in neural circuitry.

Active Components of the Musculoskeletal System

Muscle contraction is an active force of movement. A muscle must be able to generate enough force to move the segment or limb against gravity and resistance. Previously, therapists were taught that patients with neurologic damage were not weak but were hypertonic, hyper-reflexic, and bound by abnormal synergies (Craik 1991, p. 159). Changes in muscle tissue after neurologic damage have been documented. These changes include atrophy in motor units, more easily fatigued motor units, and the presence of apparently denervated muscle fibers (Dietz et al. 1986; Edström et al. 1973; Spaans and Wilts 1982). Clinical research suggests muscle weakness *is* present after neurologic insult. Gate et al. (1986), Kramer and MacPhail (1994), and Vaughn (1989) suggest that patients with neurologic damage have isometric strength in some parts of, but not throughout, the range of motion.

Muscle force, torque, and power can be quantified. Force is the product of mass and acceleration. Torque is the product of the force occurring across a joint and the perpendicular distance between the line of action of the force and the axis of joint rotation. Power is the product of torque and angular velocity of the joint. Power is generated in concentric (shortening) contractions and absorbed in eccentric (lengthening) contractions. These principles quantify forces of muscle and gravity on limb motion as well as the effect of motion of one segment on another segment.

Force, torque, and power provide quantifiable data that can be applied to analysis of motion. Because the specifics of rigid body analysis are beyond the scope of this text, the reader is referred to Schneider and Zernicke (1990) for an in-depth examination. This dynamic analysis provides insight into different conditions of motor control that may produce the same kinematics. For example, a joint may flex from the action of either a concentric flexion force or an eccentric extensor force. Applied to therapy, strengthening the hip flexor may be beneficial if the motion is due to a concentric flexor force such as lifting the leg to climb a step but counterproductive if the motion is due to an eccentric extensor force as occurs in the swing phase of gait. This approach has been applied to reach and gait as well as infant kicking. Discussion of the results of this type of analysis on reach and gait follows the insight into dynamic biomechanics gained from the analysis of the cat and infant.

The work of Hoy and Zernicke (1986), Hoy et al. (1985), and Smith and Zernicke (1987) analyzes the dynamics of a cat's paw shake. A cat's paw shake is a rapid oscillatory movement of the hip, knee, and ankle used by a cat to remove something attached to its hind paw. These researchers found that ankle muscles produce the torques to control the paw dynamics directly. During the paw shake, the knee muscles also produce torques to control the changes in force occurring at the knee caused by the ankle motion.

Schneider et al. (1990) followed with an investigation of the kicking motion of supine 3-month-old infants. The analysis was applied to kicks ranging from nonvigorous to very vigorous. The decrease in flexion occurring at the hip during the nonvigorous kick was primarily a result of gravity. The hip flexor responded to counteract the effect of gravity. The hip flexor was joined by flexor torques generated between the segments of the limb, producing motion-dependent torques (torques due to motion of other segments in a linked system). In vigorous kicking, an extensor-muscle torque appeared to counteract the flexor effect of the motion-dependent torques. In very vigorous kicking the extensor torque was also necessary to counteract the force of the hip flexor that had responded to gravity in the nonvigorous kicking. Even though the motion looked the same, the force producing the motion differed in the interaction of forces produced by muscle, motion dependence, and gravity. This could explain why, in therapy, a child can produce a desired motion if practiced slowly (using a particular pattern of torques) but cannot use the motion functionally in school or home settings (because it requires a different pattern of torques).

Skill changes through practice of a particular movement, resulting in improved speed or accuracy for that movement.

Beyond task-specific skills, however, movement changes in terms of efficiency (Bernstein 1967), economy and efficiency (Cavanaugh and Kram 1985), and smoothness (Nelson 1983).

Efficiency of movement means minimizing the energy necessary to successfully accomplish a task. Hence, "ideal posture" is efficient because it minimizes the torques of gravity around the joints allowing stance with minimal muscle effort. The six determinants of gait (lateral pelvic tilt, knee flexion, knee-ankle-foot interaction, pelvic rotation, and physiologic nalgus) are responsible for lowering the energy cost of ambulation by decreasing the muscle force necessary to move the body. Therapy often focuses on improving the quality or look of a movement. A more functional goal may be improving the efficiency of movement. How many times have children been able to walk slowly with at least a flat-foot, if not a heel-toe, gait in therapy only to run out of the room at the end of therapy right back up on their toes? The child is not interested in the quality of the movement but in keeping up with peers.

Control of Reach in Adults

Zernicke and Schneider (1993) addressed the concept of smoothness. Adult subjects were asked to move the hand from a target at hip level to a target at shoulder level while avoiding a barrier. In initial stages of practice, muscular force of the shoulder flexors was necessary to overcome the effects of gravity. With practice, not only did speed increase but the muscular role changed as well, producing a smoother pattern of limb movement. Initially the shoulder flexors contracted to overcome gravity, actively slowing the shoulder flexion just before the hand reached the target. In slow trials, the shoulder muscles reached a point of co-contraction. As speed increased however, the shoulder extensors appeared significantly earlier in the motion, slowing the rate of shoulder flexion and placing the extensor on stretch. This stretched position maximizes the viscoelastic properties of the muscle, producing more force. Essentially, slower motions recruit muscle to overcome gravity whereas faster motions use muscle force to counterbalance intersegmental forces changing throughout the motion

(motion-dependent torques). An action performed slowly is not the same motion (i.e., does not involve the same muscle mechanics) as the same action performed at functional speed.

Control of Reach in Infants

Thelen et al. (1993) studied the development of infant reach. Infant reach begins as an erratic motion that becomes more coordinated (smoother or more efficient) over time. Thelen et al., in conjunction with Zernicke and Schneider (1993), have documented a change in the muscular torques (during an infant's reach) relative to gravity and the motion-dependent torques such as inertia and linear and angular acceleration. Initially (5–22 weeks of age), the infant showed an erratic pattern to generating muscle torque, consistent with his exploration of inertia and acceleration (i.e., the infant used force at both the elbow and shoulder to overcome gravity and inertia). At 30 weeks of age, the infant showed a pattern of power generation first at both the elbow and shoulder and then by a phase of power generation at the shoulder and power absorption at the elbow. In other words, the infant initially used force at both the elbow and shoulder to overcome inertia, then used the shoulder to continue to raise the limb against gravity while the elbow extended to place the hand. Finally, by 50 weeks, the infant first used muscle power at both the elbow and shoulder, followed by a phase of power absorption at the elbow and power generation at the shoulder, and lastly a phase of power absorption at both the elbow and shoulder joints. The muscle force at the elbow and shoulder was used to overcome gravity and inertia. Then the shoulder muscle force raised the arm while overcoming the added resistance of the extending arm as the elbow extended to place the hand. Zernicke and Schneider (1993) and Thelen et al. (1993) suggest that the infant initially used muscle power to move his limb segments individually but developed the ability to adjust muscle power to respond to the effects of motion-dependent torques producing coordinated reach. Thelen et al. (1993) state that

> *infants assembled reaching skill in a dynamic, context-specific fashion, using whatever components they individ-*

ually had available for the task. . . . the skills emerged from the confluence of components that were continuous and manifest: the ability to visually locate the toy in space, intention to reach and grab the toy and transport it to the mouth, growing control of the head and trunk, and the increasing ability to modulate the force and compliance of the arms (p. 1093).

Chapter 4 focuses on the last component—the ability to modulate the force and compliance of the limbs. Extra-articular connective tissue flexibility, muscle length, muscle strength, and muscle endurance are four variables that can be altered in therapy to assist the child in his or her "dynamic" and "context-specific" exploration of the "perceptual consequences of self-generated movement" (Thelen et al. 1993, p. 1094).

4

Principles of Mobilization for Neurologic Disorders

Theories of motor control stress the importance of the interaction among the nervous, skeletal, muscular, and cardiovascular systems to produce efficient movement. Imbalance in any of the systems directly impairs motor efficiency; multiple imbalances in several systems can mimic each other's effect on movement. Children with a primary neurologic insult have an initial imbalance in one system that interacts to produce imbalances in other systems as children grow.

The classic history of a child with cerebral palsy illustrates this interaction. Children with cerebral palsy are seldom diagnosed at birth even if there is a history of intraventricular bleeds. However, over time, concerns are raised regarding the limited amount of movement and the difficulty of the movement performed. Relative immobility of all systems can be seen. These effects include weakness, increased heart rate and respiratory rate with minimal exertion, thickening of the ligaments, and failure of bones to remodel to mature patterns, to name a few. Over time, the child's weakness compared to peers becomes more pronounced. With more time the skeletal system responds to the imbalance in the neurologic and muscular systems by failing to develop normally (usually at the hips) or by developing abnormally (often in the spine). Multiple imbalances in various systems interfere with the child's attempts to move. For treatment to be effective, the assessment must determine which imbalances in which systems are interfering with the child's movement.

The system-based assessment is addressed in Chapter 5. Because therapists who traditionally focused on treating clients with neurologic insults are frequently less familiar with orthopedic approaches than neurologic ones, this chapter presents an overview of orthopedic assessment including mobilization. The orthopedic assessment addresses bone growth, both in shape and alignment; joint formation; and tissue support of the joint. Principles of assessing and treating joint limitations through mobilization are then discussed.

Bone Growth

Bones grow based on stresses placed on them. These stresses include weightbearing and muscle pull. For children with neurologic damage, stresses from both weightbearing and muscle pull are changed. It is well documented that bones of children with unilateral neurologic insult grow but are smaller on the affected side than on the less affected side (Campbell 1989, LeVeau and Bernhardt 1984).

Bone formation in the child with neurologic insult begins normally. Hence, children with neurologic impairment frequently have the normal variability of internal or external femoral torsion seen in any other child. However, over time, the lack of normal stresses (e.g., muscle action at the hip) and the presence of abnormal stresses (e.g., unequal muscle pull on the spine) produce common orthopedic problems such as dislocated hips and paralytic scoliosis. Anomalous amounts of torsion in the bones may be maintained or resolved as for any other child but appear to be maintained due to limitations in supporting tissues. The orthopedic assessment discriminates between bone shape and limitations of other supporting tissues imitating anomalous bone shape.

Joint Formation

Joints form early in fetal development. Therefore, they are seldom initially deformed or limited by the neurologic damage per se.

However, the relative hypomobility or immobility subsequent to the neurologic insult can have consequences on joint formation.

The effect of immobility on joint development of the hip provides an excellent example. At birth, the hip joint is in a position of contracture due to capsular limitations (Lee 1977). Decrease in the contracture normally occurs as the hips are extended and externally rotated, when infants attempt to get their heads up in prone or are supported in standing. Because children with neurologic damage such as cerebral palsy cannot stretch their own hip connective tissue because of the accompanying muscle weakness, the normal newborn contracture tends to be maintained. The older child with neurologic damage and a hip flexion contracture may not have developed abnormal contracture but rather maintained the normal infantile contracture. Maintenance of the contracture prevents the forces of weightbearing and muscle pull to remodel the femur as the forces are applied across the wrong part of the joint. This may account for the high incidence of subluxed hips in children with neurologic damage.

Joint Support Tissues

The connective tissue surrounding a synovial joint includes the ligaments and capsule. By definition, the function of these structures is to limit excessive mobility about the joint. Immobility causes the connective tissue to tighten (Threlkeld 1992), limiting not only excessive movement but normal range of motion as well. This occurs regardless of whether the cause of the immobility is a cast placed subsequent to a fracture or to a neurologic insult and concomitant weakness. At the hip, for example, the connective tissue is normally tight at birth because of the normal relative immobility before birth (Bleck 1982; Haas et al. 1973; Hensinger and Jone 1982; Lee 1977; McCrea 1985). Postnatally, the infant kicks gradually stretch the connective tissue structures. By 3 months of age the normal congenital hip contracture of 60 degrees has been reduced to 10 degrees (Bleck 1982; Haas et al. 1973; Hensinger and Jone

1982; Hoffer 1980; McCrea 1985; Sgarlato 1971). By 9 months the contracture continues to decrease to 3 degrees. Finally, full range of adult motion is present by 2–3 years of age.

If the child has a neurologic impairment, producing weakness or in any other way interfering with force production across the hip connective tissue structures, the joint evolution is different. Because that child cannot move much, or at all, the contracture is maintained and reinforced. At first, this is not noticeable because the presence of the contracture is expected. However, as the child matures, the contracture does not resolve. The medical community usually describes this as the development of an abnormal contracture, as opposed to the maintenance of a normal infantile connective tissue contracture.

With the connective tissue contracture just described, there is a limitation in free age-appropriate range of motion at the hip joint. The ranges particularly affected are extension and external rotation. Abnormal bone formation and short muscles are usually considered causes of the limited extension and external rotation with resultant in-toeing. Although these abnormalities may be present, the connective tissue limitation by itself produces limited range of motion and the appearance of in-toeing that mimics anteverted hips. The purpose of the therapy assessment is to determine which system(s) is interfering in the child's motor performance. As the example illustrates, joint connective tissue limitations can mimic other causes of motor impairment.

Mobilization

Principles of Mobilization

Mobilization is a technique designed to stretch the articular support structures of the synovial joints. The technique involves determining which way to push the articular surface (determined from the rule of convex and concave), in what part of the range (determined from closed-pack and open-pack positions), and how

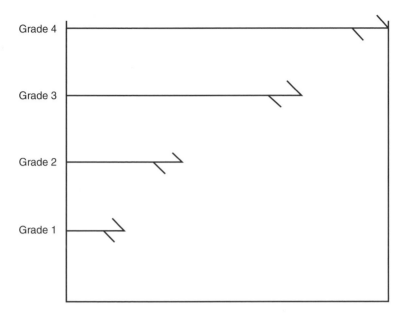

FIGURE 4-1. Total joint play available.

far to push it (determined by the grades of motion) to achieve normal joint play for normal physiologic range of motion. Each concept is addressed.

Joint Play

Accessory movements that can be passively but not actively performed at a joint are "joint play" (Kessler and Hertling 1983; Maitland 1977). These accessory movements require flexible extra-articular connective tissue to stretch across joints as the articular surfaces glide across each other. Mobilization techniques attempt to increase joint play in those synovial joints with abnormal connective tissue limitations.

Grades of Motion

To effectively stretch connective tissue structures, force is applied to varying degrees in an oscillatory pattern (Figure 4-1). Choice of grade depends on desired outcome. Grades 1 and 2 decrease joint irritability; grades 3 and 4 increase joint range of motion. In acute orthopedic conditions, grades 1 and 2 are frequently employed. In the chronic immobility associated with neurologic insults, grades 3 and 4 are usually more effective.

Closed-Pack, Open-Pack Positions

Closed-pack position of a joint describes joint surfaces that are maximally congruent, with ligaments at their most taut. This is, by definition, a stable position for the joint and occurs in the part of the range of motion where stability is required for that joint's function. Thus, for the hip joint, closed-pack occurs in full extension with adduction and in internal rotation (e.g., the position of single limb stance).

Open-pack position is any position of a joint that is not in closed-pack position. Limitation to range of motion in any part of the range other than closed-pack position suggests the possibility of ligamentous limitation. The oscillations of the grades of motion described above are applied at the point in the range where abnormal connective tissue tightness is demonstrated.

Rule of Convex and Concave

The point in the range of motion where the grades of motion are applied is determined by the connective tissue limitation found in what should be an open-pack position for the joint. The direction in which to apply the force is determined by the rule of convex and concave. The rule of convex and concave states that when a convex surface moves on a fixed concave surface, the articular surface moves in the direction opposite the shaft; when a concave surface moves on a fixed convex surface, the articular surface moves in the same direction as the shaft (Figure 4-2).

Indications and Contraindications

Mobilization is indicated when the assessment identifies connective tissue tightness as a proximate cause of limited range of motion and function. It is contraindicated when the stresses of the

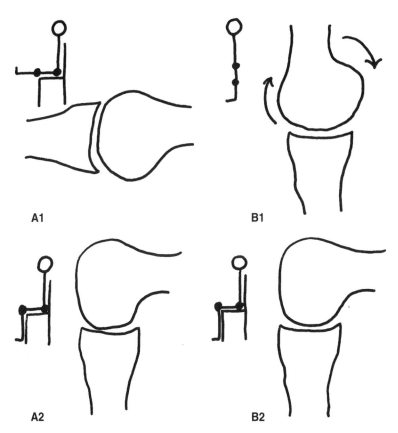

FIGURE 4-2. Rule of convex and concave as illustrated at the knee. **A.** The tibia moves on the femur to produce flexion. **B.** The femur moves on the tibia to produce flexion.

techniques cause more damage to surrounding tissues. This can occur in four types of situations:

1. Risk of fracture exists in children with a history of pathologic fractures.

2. Joint inflammation is a contraindication in children with active rheumatoid arthritis or an acute reaction to trauma.

3. Desired hypomobility can occur at the foot in a child with athetosis, at the subtalar joint (but not at the ankle joint)

subsequent to a triple arthrodesis, or in the spine after spinal fusion in spina bifida or spinal muscular atrophy.

4. Hypermobility.

Appropriate Mobilization Techniques

Children with central nervous system damage tend to have classic contractures. The classic contractures and the techniques to address them (Figures 4-3 through 4-15) if a joint limitation is a contributing cause are as follows:

1. Limited hip flexion and abduction causing sacral sitting may benefit from inferior glide of the hip.

2. Limited hip extension and abduction interfering with standing and walking may benefit from posterior-anterior glide at the hip.

3. Limited knee extension causing crouch standing and gait may benefit from posterior-anterior glide or rotary glide of the tibia.

4. Limited ankle dorsiflexion and supination/pronation causing foot deformity may benefit from anterior-posterior glide of the talus on the tibia as well as techniques for the specific deformity within the foot.

5. Limited shoulder flexion and abduction interfering with reach may benefit from elevation/protraction of the clavicle at the sternoclavicular joint or from posterior-anterior glide and inferior glide of the humerus.

6. Limited elbow extension and supination may benefit from anterior-posterior glide of the radius on the ulna.

7. Limited wrist radial deviation and extension may benefit from the combination of techniques illustrated in Figures 4-14 and 4-15.

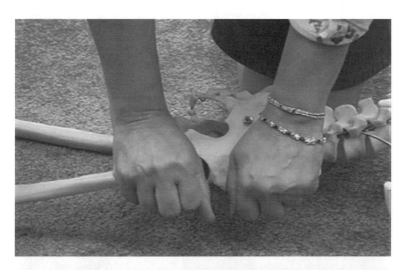

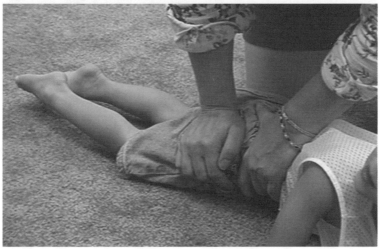

FIGURE 4-3
Technique: posterior-anterior glide of the femur.
Stabilizing hand placement: supports the anterior-superior iliac spine to prevent pelvic movement.
Mobilizing hand placement: on the posterior of the head of the femur and greater trochanter.
Direction of force: push the head of the femur anteriorly.
Purpose of the technique: to increase hip extension and external rotation.

(Reprinted with permission from S Brooks-Scott. Joint Mobilization for the Neurologically Involved Child; and Joint Mobilization for the Child with Neurological Impairment [videotapes]. Albuquerque, NM: Clinician's View, 1998.)

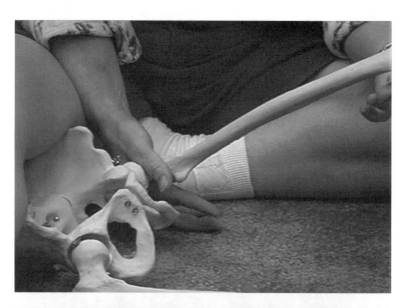

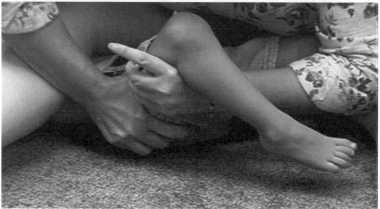

FIGURE 4-4

Technique: inferior glide of the femur.

Stabilizing hand placement: on the pelvis to prevent pelvic motion.

Mobilizing hand placement: on the femur above the greater trochanter.

Direction of force: inferior along the inguinal ligament.

Purpose of the technique: increases flexion and to a lesser extent extension and external rotation.

(Reprinted with permission from S Brooks-Scott. Joint Mobilization for the Neurologically Involved Child; and Joint Mobilization for the Child with Neurological Impairment [videotapes]. Albuquerque, NM: Clinician's View, 1998.)

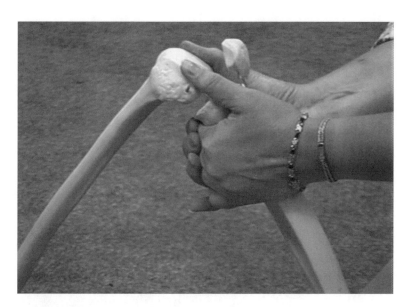

FIGURE 4-5
Technique: anterior glide of the tibia on the femur.
Stabilizing hand placement: on the distal component of the femur.
Mobilizing hand placement: on the posterior component of the tibia.
Direction of force: anteriorly in the plane of the condyles.
Purpose of the technique: increases extension of the knee from full flexion to the last 15 degrees of extension.

(Reprinted with permission from S Brooks-Scott. Joint Mobilization for the Neurologically Involved Child; and Joint Mobilization for the Child with Neurological Impairment [videotapes]. Albuquerque, NM: Clinician's View, 1998.)

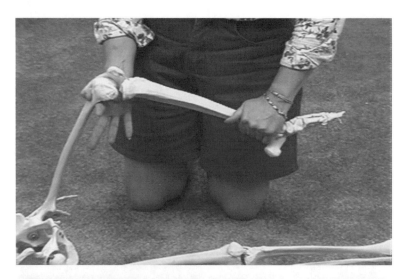

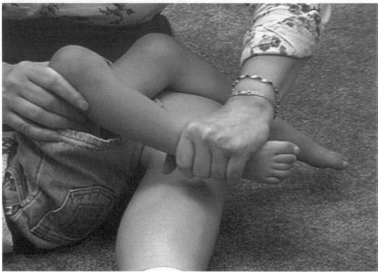

FIGURE 4-6

Technique: tibial external rotation.

Stabilizing hand placement: on the distal component of the femur.

Mobilizing hand placement: around the malleoli.

Direction of force: rotary.

Purpose of the technique: increases extension in the last 15 degrees of knee flexion.

(Reprinted with permission from S Brooks-Scott. Joint Mobilization for the Neurologically Involved Child; and Joint Mobilization for the Child with Neurological Impairment [videotapes]. Albuquerque, NM: Clinician's View, 1998.)

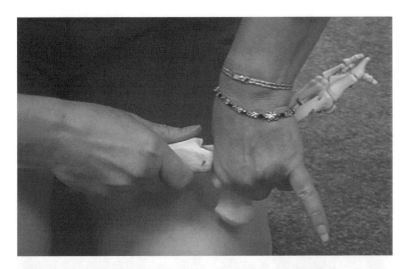

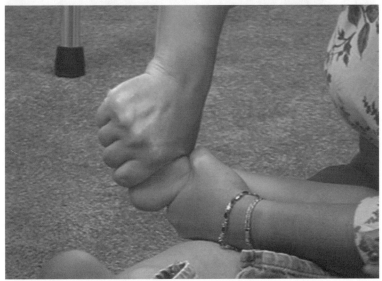

FIGURE 4-7
Technique: anterior-posterior glide of the talus.
Stabilizing hand placement: on the lower tibia and malleoli.
Mobilizing hand placement: on the web space that lies across the anterior component of the talus.
Direction of force: posterior in the plane of the talus.
Purpose of the technique: increases dorsiflexion of the talocrural joint.

(Reprinted with permission from S Brooks-Scott. Joint Mobilization for the Neurologically Involved Child; and Joint Mobilization for the Child with Neurological Impairment [videotapes]. Albuquerque, NM: Clinician's View, 1998.)

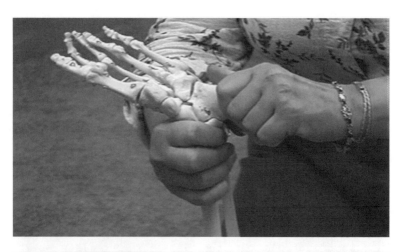

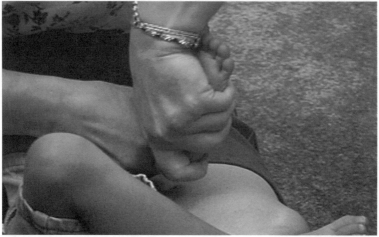

FIGURE 4-8
Technique: supination/pronation of the subtalar joint.
Stabilizing hand placement: on the distal component of the malleoli and across the talus.
Mobilizing hand placement: on the distal component of the calcaneous.
Direction of force: around a triplanar axis to increase supination/pronation; around a sagittal axis to increase inversion/eversion; around a coronal axis to increase dorsiflexion/plantar flexion; around a vertical axis to increase abduction/adduction.
Purpose of the technique: to increase supination/pronation if force applied in triplanar axis; to increase inversion/eversion if force applied across a sagittal axis; to increase dorsiflexion/plantar flexion if force applied across a coronal axis; to increase abduction/adduction if force applied across a vertical axis.

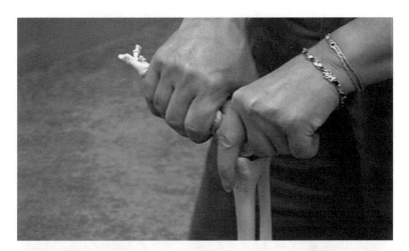

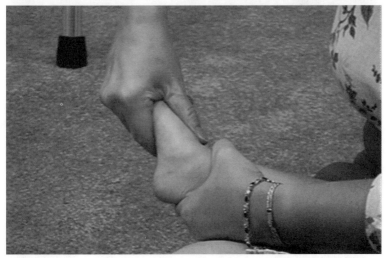

FIGURE 4-9

Technique: supination/pronation of the midtarsal joint.

Stabilizing hand placement: on the distal component of the calcaneous.

Mobilizing hand placement: on the distal component of the cuboid and navicular.

Direction of force: around a triplanar axis to increase supination/pronation; around a sagittal axis to increase inversion/eversion; around a coronal axis to increase dorsiflexion/plantar flexion; around a vertical axis to increase abduction/adduction.

Purpose of the technique: to increase supination/pronation if force applied in triplanar axis; to increase inversion/eversion if force applied across a sagittal axis; to increase dorsiflexion/plantar flexion if force applied across a coronal axis; to increase abduction/adduction if force applied across a vertical axis.

(Reprinted with permission from S Brooks-Scott. Joint Mobilization for the Neurologically Involved Child; and Joint Mobilization for the Child with Neurological Impairment [videotapes]. Albuquerque, NM: Clinician's View, 1998.)

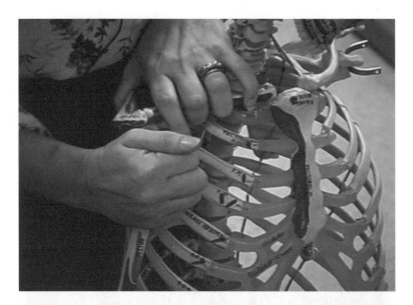

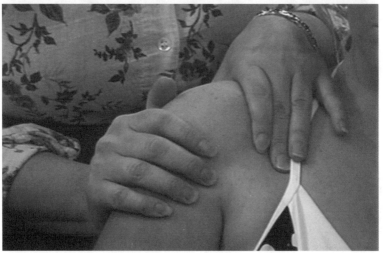

FIGURE 4-10
Technique: posterior-anterior glide of the humerus.
Stabilizing hand placement: on the clavicle and scapula.
Mobilizing hand placement: on the posterior component of the humerus.
Direction of force: anterior.
Purpose of the technique: increases external rotation of the glenohumeral joint.

(Reprinted with permission from S Brooks-Scott. Joint Mobilization for the Neurologically Involved Child; and Joint Mobilization for the Child with Neurological Impairment [videotapes]. Albuquerque, NM: Clinician's View, 1998.)

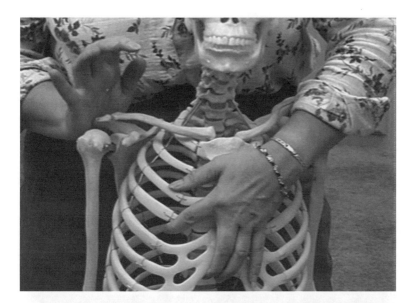

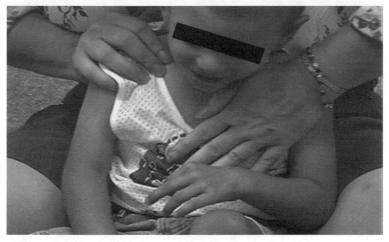

FIGURE 4-11A

Technique: sternoclavicular retraction or protraction.

Stabilizing hand placement: around the rib cage.

Mobilizing hand placement: under the inferior component of the glenoid fossa.

Direction of force: upward or forward.

Purpose of the technique: upward force increases clavicular elevation; forward force increases clavicular protraction. Both are necessary for midrange of shoulder elevation in reach.

(Reprinted with permission from S Brooks-Scott. Joint Mobilization for the Neurologically Involved Child; and Joint Mobilization for the Child with Neurological Impairment [videotapes]. Albuquerque, NM: Clinician's View, 1998.)

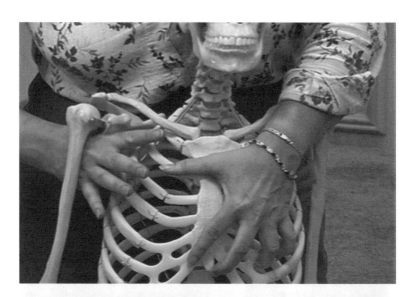

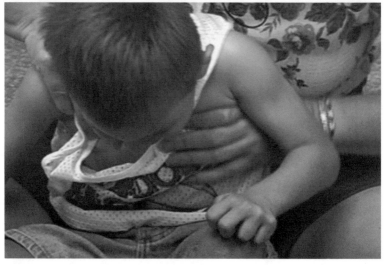

FIGURE 4-11B

Technique: sternoclavicular depression or elevation.

Stabilizing hand placement: around the rib cage.

Mobilizing hand placement: under the inferior component of the glenoid fossa.

Direction of force: upward or forward.

Purpose of the technique: upward force increases clavicular elevation; forward force increases clavicular protraction. Both are necessary for midrange of shoulder elevation in reach.

(Reprinted with permission from S Brooks-Scott. Joint Mobilization for the Neurologically Involved Child; and Joint Mobilization for the Child with Neurological Impairment [videotapes]. Albuquerque, NM: Clinician's View, 1998.)

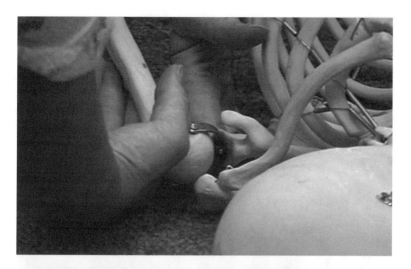

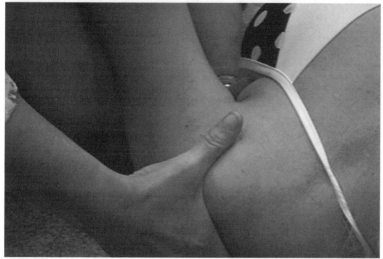

FIGURE 4-12
Technique: inferior glide of the humerus on the scapula.
Stabilizing hand placement: support the scapula to prevent sliding.
Mobilizing hand placement: on the superior component of the humerus as it protrudes from under the clavicle.
Direction of force: inferior and anterior, parallel to the surface of the glenoid fossa.
Purpose of the technique: increases shoulder flexion and abduction in the initial and terminal stages of those motions.

(Reprinted with permission from S Brooks-Scott. Joint Mobilization for the Neurologically Involved Child; and Joint Mobilization for the Child with Neurological Impairment [videotapes]. Albuquerque, NM: Clinician's View, 1998.)

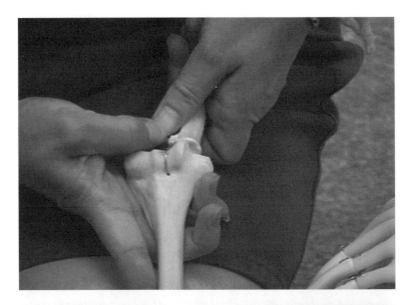

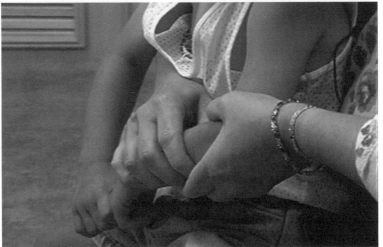

FIGURE 4-13

Technique: posterior glide of the radial head on the ulna.
Stabilizing hand placement: on the posterior aspect of the superior component of the ulna.
Mobilizing hand placement: thumbs are on the anterior aspect of the radial head.
Direction of force: posterior.
Purpose of the technique: increases elbow extension and radial ulnar supination.

(Reprinted with permission from S Brooks-Scott. Joint Mobilization for the Neurologically Involved Child; and Joint Mobilization for the Child with Neurological Impairment [videotapes]. Albuquerque, NM: Clinician's View, 1998.)

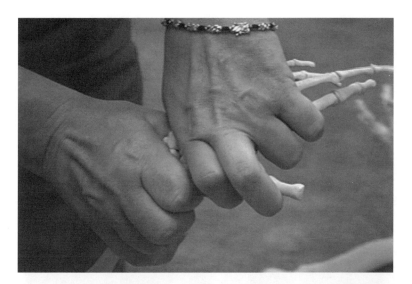

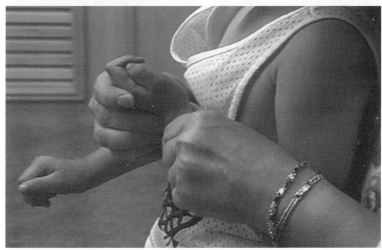

FIGURE 4-14

Technique: posterior-anterior glide of the carpals.

Stabilizing hand placement: for initial dorsiflexion, on the scaphoid; for mid-dorsiflexion, on the lunate; for terminal dorsiflexion, on the radius.

Mobilizing hand placement: for initial dorsiflexion, on the capitate; for mid-dorsiflexion, on the scaphoid; for terminal dorsiflexion, on the scaphoid.

Direction of force: for initial dorsiflexion, capitate moves palmarly; for mid-dorsiflexion, scaphoid moves dorsally; for terminal dorsiflexion, scaphoid moves palmarly.

Purpose of the technique: increases wrist extension.

(Reprinted with permission from S Brooks-Scott. Joint Mobilization for the Neurologically Involved Child; and Joint Mobilization for the Child with Neurological Impairment [videotapes]. Albuquerque, NM: Clinician's View, 1998.)

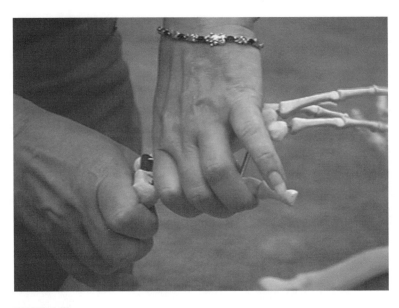

FIGURE 4-15
Technique: radial glide of the proximal carpals on the radius.
Stabilizing hand placement: on the distal component of the radius and ulna.
Mobilizing hand placement: on the proximal carpals.
Direction of force: ulnarly.
Purpose of the technique: increases radial deviation.

(Reprinted with permission from S Brooks-Scott. Joint Mobilization for the Neurologically Involved Child; and Joint Mobilization for the Child with Neurological Impairment [videotapes]. Albuquerque, NM: Clinician's View, 1998.)

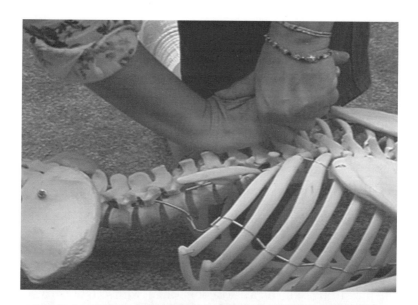

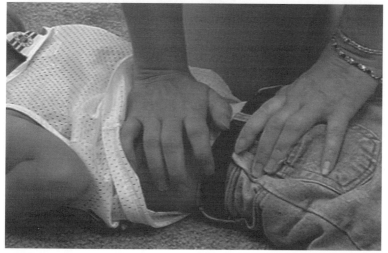

FIGURE 4-16

Technique: posterior-anterior glide of the vertebra.

Stabilizing hand placement: position the child prone. In this one technique, for this specific purpose, many joints can move.

Mobilizing hand placement: pisiform is placed over the spinous process.

Direction of force: anteriorly.

Purpose of the technique: increases mobility, especially extension, of the spine.

(Reprinted with permission from S Brooks-Scott. Joint Mobilization for the Neurologically Involved Child; and Joint Mobilization for the Child with Neurological Impairment [videotapes]. Albuquerque, NM: Clinician's View, 1998.)

Effectiveness of Mobilization

As noted, effectiveness of therapy for children with neurologic disorders is the subject of strong debate. The effectiveness of mobilization in the treatment of adult orthopedic problems is also subject to much debate. Little wonder then that Harris and Lundgren (1991) question the use of a technique that has not been well researched. As stated in the Preface, the purpose of this text is to give the reader information on which to base the discussion, formulate the questions, gather the data, and analyze the results.

Several studies of mobilization in children with neurologic disorders have been conducted. Hoesli (1989), in a single-subject study, assessed the effectiveness of inferior glide of the hip joint on the sitting skill of a 7-year-old child with cerebral palsy. Range of motion measurements were taken after the child's regular therapy sessions. The inferior glide technique was added to the regular therapy session. After 4 weeks of therapy with the additional mobilization technique, the child showed a gain of 26 degrees of hip flexion on the left and 29 degrees of hip flexion on the right. Although the range improvement is more than would be expected by measurement error, the change of sitting balance was more significant. By increasing the range of motion at the hip joints, the child's center of gravity shifted forward over the base of support, allowing the child an improved sitting balance.

Brooks (1990) reports a similar result on the sitting posture of 10 children who were sacral sitters. Similar results were found in all 10 children. The average increase in range of motion was 25 degrees. This was enough range of motion to shift the center of gravity forward, over the hips, resulting in an improved sitting balance. A similar result was reported by Brooks (1994) on a child treated by a participant in one of the mobilization seminars.

Mobilization can be a useful technique for managing motor problems in children with neurologic damage if

1. Part of the poor motor performance is due to a limitation in range of motion caused by capsular tightness.

2. Release of the capsular tightness allows freer motion or a change in the placement of the center of gravity over the base of support.

3. The child has enough understanding and motivation to use the new range of motion, enough strength to use the new range of motion functionally, and enough coordination to use the range effectively.

5

Clinical Protocols for Assessment

Heriza (1991) applies the dynamic systems approach to the assessment of children with motor dysfunction. She identifies three areas that interact and must be assessed: (1) subsystems (called *physiologic systems* in this text), (2) the physical and social environment, and (3) the task itself. Although therapists already evaluate these areas, the assumptions of our treatment frameworks and places of employment often limit the information we obtain. Heriza cites, for example, the tendency of therapists evaluating patients with neurologic impairment to focus on the nervous system. This text suggests expanding this focus to include the possible interaction of the other subsystems in movement dysfunction, as in the example of the causes of sacral sitting. Heriza points out the need to assess the subsystems of task performance. The proposed muscle strength assessment identifies age-appropriate tasks for infants and young children and determines whether children have the strength necessary to perform a given task. Finally, Heriza points out the importance of assessing the child in the environment in which the task regularly occurs. Some children move more at home or school than in the doctor's office or hospital. Architectural barriers and social-emotional stresses may vary, depending on the environment.

Heriza (1991) suggests a need to identify the collective variables, transition periods, and control parameters for each child as part of a total evaluation. Collective variables she cites include joint correlations, phase lags, and movement times. Transition periods can be identified by the variability of the movement pattern and the amount of time it takes for the pattern to return to a stable pattern after perturbation. Control parameters such as weight, height, and head circumference may be useful data. Videography, electromyography, and kinematics may be used for assessment. Although these tools are not available to the average clinician, attempts to apply the concepts of dynamic systems in the clinic can be made. For example, in gait assessment, step length, stride length, and velocity can be measured in the clinic, school, or home. Most therapy encourages children to slow down and walk with improved "quality," often at the cost of efficiency. Encouraging the child to walk at his or her own speed allows interlimb dependencies, gravity, and momentum to contribute to the motion.

Regardless of the theoretical perspective, therapy is based on an assessment of the patient. It is critical to remember that an assessment of the patient is not a theoretical construct applied to the patient. No one theory is appropriate to all patients of any diagnostic group.

The assessment approaches designed for given theoretical perspectives tend to lead the assessment of applicable aspects of the theory, but they do not suggest other theories or alternative treatment strategies (Horak 1991). On the other hand, an assessment that is independent of a treatment theory provides data from which the therapist can interpret and determine which theoretical approach(es) is appropriate. A systems approach to assessment is precisely that: a documentation of the state of a given system at the time of the assessment. If range of motion is limited, the skeletal assessment identifies the limited active range but does not immediately suggest the treatment for the problem; specific treatment approaches often do (e.g., limited range of motion is due to hypertonicity, therefore reduce tone; or limited range of motion is due to muscle tightness, therefore stretch/cut the muscle). Completion of the system assessment may find that the connective tissue surrounding the joint has limited flexibility, the muscle is too short or too weak, or the bone is misshapen. If a systems approach is used to rule out first bone anomalies, then capsular limitations, then muscle flexibility issues, and finally muscle strength issues, treatment proceeds in an efficient manner by addressing and then ruling out the specific systems contribution as a cause of the limitation of the desired motor skill. Techniques appropriate to the neurologic perspective can then be used with minimal interference from abnormalities in other systems.

As an illustration of this, consider the sacral sitting example in Chapter 4. This motor task illustrates the ability of one system to mimic dysfunction in another system. Sacral sitting is the preferred pattern of sitting for many children with cerebral palsy. In this task, the child's center of gravity is shifted to the posterior, as if the child was sitting on his or her sacrum. The difficulty of sacral sitting is that the child cannot shift his or her weight forward to balance or reach. Figure 5-1 illustrates the difference in sitting postures. Compare sacral sitting with normal sitting: In normal sitting, the center of gravity is forward of the hips and mobility is present to balance or reach forward, backward, or sideways. Table 5-1 compares the system requirements for normal sitting against the system limitations often occurring in sacral sitting.

This example suggests therapy through mobilization before reassessing the active range of motion. The reassessment may find continued limited range with increased connective tissue flexibility, yet *limited muscle strength*. Thus, strengthening, not stretching, may be in order. On the other hand, the reassessment may find *limited muscle flexibility* suggesting stretching, not strengthening, as appropriate therapy. The therapist may use orthopedic techniques, neurologic techniques, play activities, or sports activities to achieve any or all of these objectives (increased range, flexibility, and strength for more appropriate sitting). Exactly which therapeutic technique the therapist uses to achieve these ends is immaterial as long as the technique is effective. For some children, dance or participation in age-appropriate preschool activities may be equally (or more) effective than participation in twice-a-week therapy sessions. Other children may need the specific one-on-

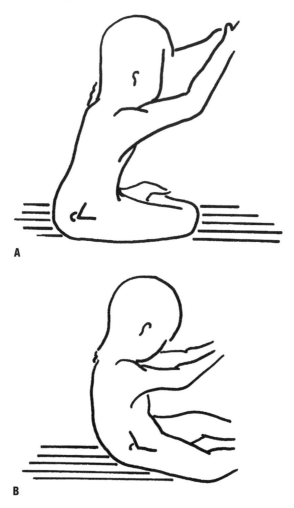

A

B

FIGURE 5-1. Functional tailor sitting **(A)** versus sacral sitting **(B)**.

one activities of a therapy session before they are able to benefit from community activities. Other children may not benefit from either. All of these possibilities must be considered in the assessment and treatment planning process.

Interpretation of the assessment in children must also take into account the normal development for the age of the child. Tables 5-2

Table 5-1. Comparison of the System Requirements for Sacral Sitting and Tailor Sitting

System	Sacral Sitting	Tailor Sitting
Skeletal		
Bone alignment		
Joint contribution	Hip capsule may limit flexion greater than 90 degrees.	Hip flexion needed for functional sitting is 120 degrees.
Muscular		
Flexibility	Hamstrings may limit hip flexion during knee extension but will not limit hip flexion during knee flexion. Does child sacral sit when the knee is flexed?	Because normal hamstring flexibility is less than 90 degrees hip flexion with the knee extended, it is normal to have a sacral sit position during periods of long sitting.
Strength	Isometric strength of the abdominals and hip flexors are needed to sacral sit.	Eccentric and concentric strength of the back extensors and hamstrings are needed to reach in tailor sitting.
Neurologic		
Shift between flexors and extensors	Because the center of gravity never moves forward of the hip joint, a child does not need to quickly shift from flexors to extensors.	As child moves back and forth in tailor sitting, the center of gravity moves forward and backward over the hip joints, requiring quick contraction and relaxation between the flexors and extensors.

and 5-3 present documented and theoretical norms for different systems' development. Note that although traditional theory suggests a skill appears when the nervous system matures, it is equally valid to suggest that skill appears when the range and strength are available to express it. All three systems (nervous, muscular, and skeletal) must be interacting before the behavior can be expressed.

Table 5-2. Normal Range of Motion Values for Children

Joint	Age (months)	Motion	Range (degrees)
Hip	0–3	Flexion	120
		Extension	−28
		Abduction	—
	3–6	Flexion	120
		Extension	−7
		Abduction	76
	9–12	Flexion	120
		Extension	−3
		Abduction	59
	18–36 (consistent with adult values)	Flexion	120
		Extension	30
		Abduction	45
Knee	0–3	Flexion	135
		Extension	Connective tissue contracture of 20–30 degrees
	6–9 (consistent with adult values)	Flexion	135
		Extension	Full hamstring and joint flexibility present by 8 mos
Shoulder	36 (not close to the adult value of 170)	Abduction: Frontal plane	90–135
		Plane of scapula	107–115
Wrist	18–36	Palmar flexion	80
		Dorsiflexion	70
		Radial deviation	20
		Ulnar deviation	30

The assessment identifies the strengths and weaknesses of the motor behavior of the child and provides documentation for the decision to enter or exit therapy. The system assessment provides an objective documentation of the needs of the child and the requirements of each system. Add the natural course of the disorder; the

Table 5-3. Proposed Functional Strength Criteria for Children*

Age (months)	Hip	Knee	Ankle	Shoulder	Trunk
3	Feet to mouth; swimming	Prone kicking; wiggles legs while sitting on someone's lap	Wiggles feet anti-gravity	Thrusts arms in play; prone "push-ups"	Feet to mouth; head steady in vertical
6	Stepping; sitting independently	—	—	Pull to sit	Turns from back to side
9	Moves from sitting to creeping or standing	Moves from sitting to creeping	—	Raises self to standing with arms	—
12	Walking, sits down with control	Sits down	Weight shifts	—	—
24	Walks up stairs	Walks up and down stairs	Squats; jumps	Throws a ball; feeds self using utensils	—
36	Kicks a ball	Kicking	Heel-toe gait appears	—	Lifts inferior angle of scapula off support in sit-up
60	—	—	—	—	Lift head and shoulder 90 degrees in sit-up

*Activities suggesting normal values for the respective ages are listed.

prognosis of the child; and the perspective of the goals of the family, educational system, and medical system, and a plan to manage the movement needs of the child can be developed. Such a plan allows criteria for entering and exiting, and possibly re-entering, therapy as well as goals for the individual intervention sessions. It also helps prevent unrealistic expectations by family and therapists and prevents therapy from becoming a guilt-release or baby-sitting session. It is important to think about therapy in light of the naturally occurring therapeutic activities available in life and the time constraints of the child. The assessment documentation, natural course of the disorder, and prognosis form the base of exit and entrance criteria discussed in Chapter 7.

6

Clinical Protocols for Treatment

Chapter 5 presented a systems approach to assessment. From that assessment comes an identification of the objective (not the goal) of therapy. The goal is the functional movement in its environment, whereas the objective of the treatment is the correction of the deficit(s) identified in one or more systems. For example, if the assessment identifies limited range of motion, the objective of the therapy session is to increase the range so the goal of age-appropriate sitting can be achieved. Tables 6-1 through 6-4 identify the limited range of motion and objectives for the relative systems of the hip and knee in stance; the hip, back, and shoulder in reach; the wrist and hand in grasp; and the foot in stance and gait.

The tables provide a comparison of normal findings and common deviations for each system in children with neurologic disorders. The system assessment allows the therapist to identify deviations from normal. Adjustment of those deviations becomes the objective. How the deviations are managed (i.e., which theoretical approach a therapist uses to achieve the objective) is a matter of individual choice, training, and skill. One reason each approach can claim eventual success is they frequently provide different means to the same end. The question for research is not which theoretical approach is better, but does the therapeutic intervention make a change in the physiologic system and ultimately improve the efficiency of the child's movement.

Seven case examples are presented in this chapter with assessment, treatment, and outcomes. As discussed in Chapter 5, many possible causes exist for the same motor behavior. Of the seven examples here, two children did not need therapy (SI and HS), three

Table 6-1. Comparison of the System Requirements for Hip and Knee in Stance

System	"Ideal" Posture	Crouch Stance
Skeletal		
Joint contribution	Hip extension of 5 degrees allows closed-pack position and placement of center of gravity behind axis of hip joint. Knee is in last 5 degrees of extension.	Hip capsule may limit extension >0 degrees with placement of center of gravity forward of hip joint, requiring muscle force to maintain position. Knee capsule may limit knee extension to −15 degrees, requiring more muscle force to control.
Muscular		
Flexibility	Hip flexors must allow joint to move into extension. Hamstring flexibility is not an issue.	Once joint flexibility is obtained, hip flexors may be tight. Hamstring flexibility is not an issue.
Strength	Eccentric and concentric strength of the flexors and extensors is used in terminal extension.	Isometric strength of the hamstrings and quads is used in excessive flexion.
Endurance	Phasic activity.	Requires sustained contraction.
Neurologic		
Shift between flexors and extensors	Phasic shifts between flexors and extensors at the end range.	Isometric contractions in 20 degrees of hip flexion prevent any shifts between flexors and extensors.

needed minimal therapy (CA, NY, and RS) and two needed ongoing therapy (JB and JG). The assessment for three of the children (JB, NY, and JG) suggested mobilization was appropriate treatment. One child (CA), who had been expected to have joint tightness, did not show capsular restriction on the assessment. In these cases, the Mobility sections include locomotion, architectural barriers, assistive devices, transfers, and transportation; the Activities of Daily Living sections include eating, dressing, and hygiene; and the Education/Play Activities sections include interaction with the envi-

Table 6-2. Comparison of the System Requirements for Shoulder in Reach

System	Reach in Tailor Sitting	Reach in Sacral Sitting
Skeletal		
Joint contribution	Hip flexion needed for functional reach in sitting is 120 degrees. Back extension through the lumbar spine. Sternoclavicular (SC) joint mobility required above 60 degrees.	Hip capsule may limit flexion >90 degrees. Lumbar extension may prevent upper trunk placement. Glenohumeral joint tightness if reach is limited to <60 degrees. SC joint tightness if reach is limited above 60 degrees.
Muscular		
Flexibility	Flexibility of abdominals, shoulder extensors.	The abdominals may be shortened with the extensors overstretched.
Strength	Strength of back extensors must include antigravity and resistance of the long lever of the arm and any weight (e.g., toy) held in hand. Shoulder muscles need antigravity strength for both long lever (i.e., elbow extension) and weightbearing (e.g., holding toy).	Back extensors often overstretched and too weak to hold lever of the trunk and head without substituting (e.g., hyperextending neck, shortening length of head and trunk). Shoulder muscles often not able to lift resistance of long lever of arm (i.e., elbow extended).
Neurologic	Rapid control of eccentric and concentric contractions, use of momentum and limb interdependencies.	Usually tonic contractions.

ronment and materials. Chapter 7 discusses the exit and entrance criteria, applying the criteria to these examples.

Case 1: CA

History

CA was a 5-year-old child of normal intelligence with spina bifida. He walked with quad canes for 20 feet in therapy but

Table 6-3. Comparison of the System Requirements for Wrist and Hand in Grasp

System	Closed-Pack for Grasp	Ulnar Deviation, Wrist Flexion
Skeletal		
Joint contribution	Capitate in closed-pack position on the scaphoid and scaphoid in closed-pack position on lunate produce slight extension and radial deviation.	Capitate often subluxed on scaphoid or stuck on scaphoid in palmar flexion.
Muscular		
Flexibility	Balanced flexibility of flexors and extensors allows intrinsic control of force at the wrist.	Imbalance of muscle length altering the length tension relationships in the muscles.
Strength	Balanced eccentric and concentric strength.	Altered length tension relationships, isometric contractions.
Neurologic		
Quickly shift between flexors and extensors	Rapid phasic motion across axes of the joints.	Usually tonic co-contraction.

primarily used a wheelchair. He wore knee-ankle-foot orthoses all the time. He went to therapy at the local hospital 1–3 days per week since birth. He did not yet attend school. He lived with his family on a private street with minimal traffic. His friends lived within three blocks of his house in the same subdivision.

Primary Concerns

The mother was concerned about her child's community ambulation such as walking from the parking lot to the library, his maintenance of range of motion, and potential problems associated with growth and the tethered cord.

Review of Systems

Orthopedic

Bone: CA had subluxed hips that had not progressed in 3 years. Surgery to correct his tethered cord was undertaken 1 year ago. His spine was fused at the level of the spina bifida.

Table 6-4. Comparison of the System Requirements for Foot in Gait

System	Stance through Push-Off	Support in Cerebral Palsy
Skeletal		
Bone alignment	At heel-strike, the talus glides medially and the subtalar joint pronates; at mid-stance, the joints move to neutral; and at push-off, the subtalar joint supinates.	Generally the foot is a rigid lever or collapses with little to no movement relative to the phases of gait.
Joint contribution	—	Hypermobility or hypomobility and malalignment are common.
Muscular		
Flexibility	—	One cannot distinguish between tightness of the gastrocnemius soleus; one can only assess when subtalar joint is properly aligned.
Strength	Eccentric and concentric contractions of flexors and extensors with balanced synergy for inversion and eversion.	Subtalar pronation shifts the axis of the gastrocnemius and tibialis muscles from supinators to pronators. Isometric contractions generally occur.
Neurologic		
Shift between flexors and extensors	Normal cadence is 150–170 steps/minute (75–85 steps/minute per limb) depending on age.	Minimal shifts between eccentric and concentric contractions, certainly not anywhere near 75–85 times/minute per limb.

Joint and support structures: CA had full range of motion at all joints with the exception of hip contractures of less than 10-degree hip flexion on the right and a 5-degree knee flexion on the left. Capsular flexibility was normal.

Muscular

Flexibility: Hip flexors and left hamstring were mildly limited as noted by the range of motion above.

Strength: CA had age-appropriate strength in the upper extremities. Hip flexors could contract against gravity through part of the range with no substitution. Hamstrings could flex the knee through part of the range, with gravity eliminated. Quadriceps could extend the knee through part of the range against gravity. No ankle muscle contractions could be palpated.

Endurance: CA walked around the gym five times in a row. He could walk throughout his house with no signs of fatigue.

Neurologic

Central nervous system (awareness, cognition, cranial nerves, stiffness, motor planning, sensation): CA was tested with normal intelligence. Cranial nerves II–XII were grossly intact. No evidence of hydrocephalus was found. Lower extremities were flaccid. CA had little to no sensation in the lower extremities from dermatome L1 down. There were no concerns regarding motor planning.

Mobility

Although CA could walk with his canes at home and at the hospital, he was not a community ambulator. Although he could ascend and descend the four steps at the hospital therapy department, he could neither ascend nor descend the 12 steps to the family room.

Activities of Daily Living

CA was independent in all activities of daily living (ADLs) except getting in and out of the bathtub.

Task Analysis

Stretching was necessary to maintain flexibility in the hip flexors and hamstring. CA had not had the opportunity to attempt truly functional walking.

Environmental Considerations

The steps at CA's home were significantly different from the steps in the hospital: They were much longer and had no guide rail. His home was on a private street with few hills. His friends lived within three blocks of his home. The sidewalks were in good condition throughout the neighborhood.

Entrance Criteria

CA had a motor problem that was a combination of sensorimotor (muscle flexibility and peripheral neural damage) and environmental (no opportunity for functional community walks) in origin. The therapist needed to assure the family that CA was up to the challenge of community walks and ascending/descending the stairs. However, the family could help alleviate the sensorimotor aspects of the problem.

Treatment Plan

Treatment focused on stretching the tight muscles and rewarding CA for attempting, then completing, the motor tasks. The therapist and CA chose the goal for the day. When the goal was accomplished the therapy session was over. This was a strong motivating factor for CA, as he was tired of therapy.

Results

CA was discharged 8 weeks later. He was able to independently ambulate with his canes to his friend's house, from the parking lot to (and through) a toy store, and from the parking lot into (and through) the library. Annual reviews were approved by the insurance company and provided to the mother when requested. When a specific need was identified, the insurance company approved additional therapy.

Exit Criteria

Goal was met.

Case 2: SI

History

SI was a 15-year-old adolescent with a diagnosis of developmental delay and an IQ of 50. She attended a self-contained classroom. Her academic program focused on functional community mobility and work skills.

Primary Concerns

Her mother wanted SI to have weekly therapy to improve SI's coordination and for general conditioning.

Review of Systems

Orthopedic

Bone: SI's hips were seated. Her spine was straight, with no evidence of scoliosis or kyphosis.

Joint and support structures: SI had active movement through the full range of motion at all joints.

Muscular

Flexibility: SI had full muscular flexibility in all major muscle groups.

Strength: SI was able to move all body parts against gravity and resistance, consistent with her daily activities. She could lift and carry laundry, perform cleaning tasks, and participate in all job-related tasks in her job-training program.

Endurance: Her mother was concerned because SI was tired after school. SI would sit and watch television until dinner.

Neurologic

Central nervous system (awareness, cognition, cranial nerves, sensory discrimination, stiffness, motor planning): SI was aware of her surroundings. Her IQ was tested at 50. Cranial nerves II–XII appeared to be intact. SI could discriminate between hot and cold, sharp and dull. No abnormal stiffness was present. Her motor planning performance was consistent with that of her peers.

Peripheral nervous system (deep tendon reflexes [DTRs], sensation): DTRs were +2.

Mobility

SI was independently ambulatory. She could maneuver around all architectural barriers in her school and work site. She could get on and off the bus independently. She used no assistive devices.

Activities of Daily Living

SI was independent in feeding, dressing, and cleaning herself.

Education/Play Activities

Activities included interaction with environment and materials. SI had difficulty using calculators with small buttons and telephones with standard buttons. She had no difficulty with door knobs or utensils.

Task Analysis

The main difficulty identified was difficulty with small buttons. Large-button phones and calculators are readily available.

Entrance Criteria

The mother was primarily concerned about SI's general conditioning and coordination necessary to use the calculator and telephone. Although these problems did or potentially will interfere with SI's success in life, they are not primarily sensorimotor based. Solutions other than therapy, including modifying the calculator and telephone and enrolling the child in a physical activity she enjoys, are more appropriate.

Treatment Plan

No treatment was recommended.

Case 3: JB

History

JB was a 3-year-old child with spastic quadriplegic cerebral palsy. He received therapy at the hospital twice a week from age 6 months to 2 years. His uncooperative behavior and outbursts (he bit his hospital-based therapist) led to twice-weekly home therapy visits. He received therapy at home for 6 months, at which time he independently ambulated with quad canes.

Primary Concerns

JB's mother was primarily concerned that he be independently mobile, as he was a very tall child and was therefore difficult to carry.

Review of Systems
Orthopedic

Bone: JB's hips were seated. His spine was straight, with no evidence of scoliosis or kyphosis.

Joint and support structures: JB's range of motion was limited at all joints as follows: Shoulder flexion was 60 degrees; elbow extension was −10 degrees; 80 degrees of hip flexion was present, whereas hip extension was −20 degrees; knees had 20-degree flexion contractures; ankle lacked 10 degrees of neutral. Capsular flexibility was limited in most joints.

Muscular

Flexibility: Muscle flexibility was present through the available joint range of motion but had to be reassessed as the joints gained flexibility. Once they had flexibility, muscular limitations were found in the hamstrings, heel cords, and adductors.

Strength: JB was able to move his limbs through part of the available range against gravity. In gravity-eliminated positions, he still had difficulty moving his hips, knees, and ankles through the full range.

Endurance: JB could stiffen and throw a tantrum for more than an hour. However, once functional movement was obtained, he exhibited muscle tremors in the calves and hamstrings after just five to six repetitions of muscle contractions.

Neurologic

Central nervous system (awareness, cognition, cranial nerves, sensory discrimination, stiffness, motor planning): JB was very aware of his surroundings even though he refused to speak or interact with anyone other than his mother. He was significantly delayed in fine and gross motor skills secondary to the cerebral palsy. JB's receptive language appeared to be age-appropriate. Self-help skills were limited by his motor impairment.

Cranial nerves II–XII appeared to be grossly intact. Sensation and motor planning could not be tested.

Peripheral nervous system (DTRs, sensation): JB's DTRs were +4 bilaterally.

Mobility

JB was totally dependent on his caregiver for all mobility. He had ankle-foot orthoses (AFOs), which he could not wear as they were molded to 90 degrees at the ankle and he only had −10 degrees of dorsiflexion.

Activities of Daily Living

JB was totally dependent.

Task Analysis

To ambulate, JB needed more joint flexibility, more muscle flexibility, and more muscle strength. A behavioral change was also necessary.

Environmental Considerations

JB lived in a small house. The distance from his room to the living room was only 20 feet. There was no furniture in his way, but he had to navigate two turns. There were no steps in either the home or the path leading from his home to his grandmother's home next door.

Entrance Criteria

JB had a motor problem that interfered with his ability to function in his world. The problem was both sensorimotor and behavioral in origin. Therapy could potentially change the motor problem as long as the behavioral problem was addressed at the same time.

Treatment Plan

JB's treatment involved a multifaceted plan, including mobilization, stretching, strengthening, and ambulation. The behavioral plan included rewards for accomplishing goals and convincing JB to set his own goals. Initially, JB was rewarded by ending therapy after completing a required task. If JB completed the task in 2 hours, he was in therapy for 2 hours. If he completed the task in 5 minutes, he was in therapy for 5 minutes. It did not take JB long to figure out how to end therapy sessions. As he began to participate in this program, the tasks and goals were increased. The extensions were not to fill the therapy hour but to achieve independent ambulation with a walker.

Results

Six months later, JB was able to independently ambulate with his walker from his room to his grandmother's house.

Exit Criteria

JB met his goal. It was unlikely that he would be able to ambulate without the walker. Direct therapy was discontinued. JB was seen on a consultative schedule as he grew.

Case 4: HS

History

HS was 6 years old. He was diagnosed with developmental delay. He attended a preschool where he received physical, occupational, and speech therapy each twice a week. He has attended the school since he was 3 years old and received home therapy services for 2½ years before that. The physical therapist insisted that HS wear a weighted jacket because he fell often. His records indicate that he was tested using standardized tests at 2½, 4, and 6 years of age. Each time he showed approximately a 50% delay in all areas.

Concerns

His mother insisted that therapy continue over the summer so that HS did not regress. The weighted jacket was worn and needed to be replaced.

Review of Systems

Orthopedic

Bone: HS's hips were seated. His spine was straight, with no signs of scoliosis or kyphosis.

Joint and support structures: HS had full range of motion actively and passively at all joints.

Muscular

Flexibility: Muscle flexibility was normal in all major muscle groups.

Strength: Muscle strength appeared in the normal range for age; HS could raise body parts against gravity with age-appropriate resistance.

Endurance: HS could play all day and perform repetitive tasks with no evidence of fatigue.

Neurologic

Central nervous system (awareness, cognition, cranial nerves, sensory discrimination, stiffness, motor planning): HS was aware of his surroundings. He exhibited consistent delays in self-help, fine and gross motor, speech, and language skills. He had been repeatedly tested over the last 6 years, consistently showing an approximately 50% delay in all areas. Cranial nerves II–XII appeared to be grossly intact. No abnormal stiffness was noted. HS had difficulty performing novel movements; he required extensive repetition of directions.

Peripheral nervous system (DTRs, sensation): HS could discriminate hot and cold, sharp and dull. He could tell if and where he had been touched.

Mobility

HS could walk, run, and climb. According to the therapist, teacher, and mom, he fell "a lot." When data was requested documenting how often he fell and on what surfaces, none could be produced. On observation of the child on the playground, he was able to keep up with his 6-year-old peers, although his skill was more comparable with the preschoolers in the next playground. He was not observed to fall more than any other child.

Task Analysis

Without data on how often the child fell with and without the jacket, it is impossible to tell if the jacket was any benefit to the child. Although his motor skills were not commensurate with his 6-year-old peers, they were proportionate with his overall development.

Entrance Criteria

Although the problem of falling interfered with his ability to participate in his environment according to the therapist, his teacher, and his mom, no data supported that conclusion. This problem did not appear to be primarily sensorimotor based, as many other explanations are available for the performance and few deficits in the physiologic systems. It is unlikely that this child benefited from 6 years of therapy considering his progress was consistent throughout. It is undocumented that the weighted jacket was of any benefit. Given that it is 90+ degrees in the summer where this child lives, a weighted jacket was potentially more hindrance than help.

Treatment Plan

No services were recommended for the summer.

Results

The child showed no more lack of skills than any other child returning to school in the fall.

Case 5: RS

History

RS is a 3-year-old boy. He was born 2 weeks postmature. He was diagnosed with congenital dislocated hips for which he wore a Pavlik harness. He appeared to be developing normally until 5 months of age, when he was hospitalized for respiratory syncytial virus. Within the month he developed left-leg weakness followed rapidly by right-leg, trunk, and upper-extremity weakness.

Within a few days he could not cough. He was hospitalized with a diagnosis of Guillain-Barré syndrome. He began intravenous immunoglobulin treatment. After a year of gradual progression of weakness, he was retested. Biopsy and genetic testing confirmed the new diagnosis of spinal muscular atrophy, type 1.

Primary Concerns

On the medicine, RS was not showing the usual rapid progression of weakness. In fact, he gradually improved and stabilized. He was a gifted child with minimal mobility. He could not roll but could sit with support. He could use a track-ball mouse to play games on the computer. He could also feed himself with a spoon, drink from a straw, and drink from a cup (if less than 4 oz of fluid were in the cup). His mother's concern was that he be as independent as possible.

Review of Systems

Orthopedic

Bone: RS's hips were dislocated. He had a 45-degree scoliosis.
Joint and support structures: RS had full passive, but not active, range of motion at all joints including his hips.

Muscular

Flexibility: RS had limited flexibility of his gastrocnemius soleus to approximately –5 degrees of dorsiflexion.

Strength: RS was able to move through part of the range of motion with gravity eliminated at all major joints. He was able to move through part of the range of motion against gravity at his knees and right shoulder. He was able to move through the full range against gravity with a little resistance at his elbows and hands.

Endurance: RS fatigued after playing for approximately 1 hour. His increased difficulty in moving his arms or hands to continue playing his games confirmed this.

Neurologic

Central nervous system (awareness, cognition, cranial nerves, sensory discrimination, stiffness, motor planning): RS was very aware of his surroundings. His gross and fine motor and self-help skills were scored at the 0- to 3-month-old level on standardized tests. His language scores were at a 5-year-old level. Cranial nerves appeared to be intact. He was able to discriminate between hot and cold, sharp and dull. He was flaccid.

Peripheral nervous system (DTRs, sensation): His DTRs were 0.

Mobility

RS had a manual wheelchair. He lived in a two-story home with two steps at the entrance of the house. He had a body jacket, AFOs, and a standing frame.

Activities of Daily Living

RS was essentially dependent in all self-help skills.

Education/Play Activities

RS played games on his computer for hours. He watched videos. He liked fishing, throwing balls, and playing with blocks. He was just starting preschool.

Task Analysis

To improve RS's independence, he either needed to improve his skills or adapt to the environment. Given his response to the medicine it was impossible to say whether he would make improvements, but environmental adaptation would allow independence regardless of his response to the medicine.

Environmental Considerations

RS had his own computer in a wheelchair-accessible location. The home had carpeting and wood floors. Doorways were standard widths, but there were double-wide doors between all rooms except the kitchen.

Entrance Criteria

His problems certainly interfered with his ability to interact with his environment; his problems were primarily sensorimotor based. Potential to change had to be considered when determining whether he would change or adapt to his environment.

Treatment Plan

RS received therapy two times per week over the past year. He has shown improvement in his strength as noted above. He has entered preschool. His mother is suggesting less therapy, more time with a teacher for the gifted, and an adapted-technology consultant.

Results

The school has agreed to provide therapy twice a week, a visit by the teacher once a month, and a consult with the adaptive technology specialist.

Case 6: NY

History

NY was a 3-year-old child with spastic diplegia. She had been receiving therapy since she was 6 months old. For 6 months, she had been able to ambulate for two to three steps, but then would fall. She received fixed-ankle AFOs 1 month before the session. With the AFOs, she was also only able to ambulate for two to three steps before falling. She walked on her toes, whether in or out of the AFOs.

Primary Concerns

NY's ambulation was not functional. She was getting too big to be carried and was due to start school in the fall.

Review of Systems
Orthopedic

Bone: NY's hips were seated and stable. Her spine had appropriate curves, no evidence of scoliosis.

Joint and support structures: NY had full active range of motion in all major joints except the ankles. NY lacked 5 degrees of dorsiflexion bilaterally, both actively and passively. Joint performance at the ankle was lacking.

Muscular

Flexibility: Full muscle flexibility was present in all major muscle groups except the plantar flexors. The flexibility could not be tested until joint flexibility was achieved.

Strength: NY was able to move all limbs against gravity and resistance as appropriate for her age. She was not able to dorsiflex or plantar flex her feet, even in response to a tickle.

Endurance: NY was able to play by herself for extended periods, during which she was able to repeat tasks with no evidence of muscle fatigue.

Neurologic

Central nervous system (awareness, cognition, cranial nerves, sensory discrimination, stiffness, motor planning): NY was very aware of her surroundings. She exhibited age-appropriate speech, fine motor, and self-help skills. Cranial nerves II–XII were grossly intact. She could distinguish between hot and cold, sharp and dull. She exhibited increased stiffness throughout her lower extremities. She could plan and execute fine motor tasks appropriately.

Peripheral nervous system (DTRs, sensation): DTRs were +3 in the lower extremities, +2 in the upper extremities.

Mobility

She could rise and stand independently, though she did so on her toes. Mobility was as described under History.

Task Analysis

Because NY ambulated with essentially the same pattern with and without the AFOs, the braces appeared to contribute little to her mobility. Because she stood on her toes both in and out of the AFOs, they contributed little to improve her posture. Other issues that may have interfered with her gait included muscle weakness and the limited joint flexibility. Standing required approximately 5 degrees of dorsiflexion and eccentric/concentric strength of the gastrocnemius soleus group. Ambulation also requires 3–5 degrees of dorsiflexion and eccentric/concentric strength of the gastrocnemius soleus group (although through a larger range than that required for standing).

Entrance Criteria

The problems outlined certainly interfered with NY's ability to interact effectively. There is at least a sensorimotor contribution to the problem. Previous attempts have essentially not changed the motor performance. A different approach may be able to positively affect the motor problem.

Treatment Plan

Anterior-posterior glide of the talus on the tibia was tried in order to gain ankle joint flexibility and sufficient range of motion for the task. This was followed by attempts to elicit contractions of the gastrocnemius soleus group in gravity-eliminated positions.

Results

Because NY ambulated with the same pattern with or without the AFOs, they appeared to provide little benefit. An anterior-posterior glide of the ankle produced increased joint flexibility producing greater than 5 degrees of dorsiflexion bilaterally. After the increased range of motion, NY was still unable to stand independently. Her inability to control her increased dorsiflexion shifted the center of gravity too far forward, and she had to hold onto an object for stability while standing. No response of the gastrocnemius soleus group was seen in response to this stretch, to tickling, or to active attempts to present plantar flex in a gravity-eliminated position. After putting on the AFOs, NY was able to stand flat-footed while playing a game. She was able to ambulate more than 50 steps without falling.

Exit Criteria

The goal of the session had been met. The potential for further strengthening in the gastrocnemius soleus group was debatable.

Case 7: JG

History

JG was born with L4–5 spina bifida, repaired shortly after birth. She has an Arnold-Chiari malformation. She has hydrocephalus that was shunted. At the time of referral, JG was 2 years old. She was on 0.2 liters of oxygen. She had received therapy since she was stable enough to tolerate it. The previous therapy program focused on enabling JG to sit and crawl.

Primary Concerns

JG's parents expressed general concerns regarding fulfilling her potential as well as concerns regarding her overall health. Many health professionals had told them that JG would die, so they had few expectations but lots of hope.

Review of Systems

Orthopedic

Bone: JG's hips were subluxed. Her spine was straight, lacking the normal lumbar curve secondary to the spinal fusion at birth. Thoracic kyphosis had not yet appeared.

Joint and support structures: JG's range-of-motion limitations were as follows: Her hips lacked 20 degrees of extension and barely showed 90 degrees of flexion. Knees lacked 10 degrees of extension. Ankles had greater than 5 degrees of dorsiflexion. Upper extremities showed full passive shoulder flexion and abduction, but active range was limited to approximately 90 degrees. Supination was limited to neutral bilaterally. Wrists and fingers were within normal limits. All joints with limitations exhibited limits in capsular flexibility.

Muscular

Flexibility: Muscle flexibility was present through all ranges noted above, to be reassessed after capsular limitations were addressed.

Strength: JG could tilt her head from side to side and shake her head yes. She could raise her arms to approximately

90 degrees with her elbows bent and to approximately 60 degrees with her elbows straight. She could grasp an infant toy (approximately 4 oz) and bring it to her mouth, but she could not pick up age-appropriate toys because they tend to be heavier. She moved her legs very little. She could not raise her legs with antigravity in supine, though she could hold them, if placed there. She could straighten the knees and hips when supported on the floor in a supine position. She could dorsiflex her ankles through part of the range on the left and through all of the range on the right.

Endurance: JG could repeat most movements more than 10 times when she was interested in the task. She had difficulty repeating left ankle dorsiflexion more than five to six times.

Neurologic

Central nervous system (awareness, cognition, cranial nerves, sensory discrimination, stiffness, motor planning): JG was aware of her surroundings. She liked toys that made noise or had bright colors. Although she is too young for formal cognitive testing, her speech and language, fine and gross motor, and social adaptive skills were all significantly delayed. Cranial nerves II–XII appeared grossly intact. She had not shown evidence of discrimination between hot and cold or sharp and dull. Lower extremities tended to be flaccid, consistent with the lower motor neuron damage. Upper extremities did not show evidence of increased stiffness, DTRs, or clonus.

Peripheral nervous system (DTRs, sensation): JG could respond to touch and tickle on the trunk and upper extremities. She did not appear to respond to touch along any of the lumbar or sacral dermatomes. DTRs were absent in the lower extremities and +1 in the upper extremities.

Cardiovascular

Respiratory rate at rest and on exertion: JG was on oxygen at rest.

Heart rate at rest and on exertion: JG's heart rate was erratic, and she was usually on a monitor.

Mobility

JG lived in a split-level home. She was transported in a standard child's stroller or carried. She had no assistive devices.

Activities of Daily Living

JG was dependent on assistance in all ADLs including feeding herself. She had no difficulty chewing or swallowing but had difficulty feeding herself, even finger feeding.

Education/Play Activities

JG could play with small toys by mouthing or spinning them, though her attention to them was short. She preferred watching television or interacting with people.

Task Analysis

JG's assessment suggested self-feeding and mobility as two tasks to be addressed. Her parents were in agreement.

Environmental Considerations

JG had a nurse 16 hours per day. The person filling the position changed frequently, sometimes on a daily basis. Consequently, many caregivers were available for both feeding and mobility practice, but they would have to be trained in the program established for JG. Concerns regarding mobility included navigating a stairwell, furniture in the narrow hallway leading to her bedroom, and the oxygen tubing.

Entrance Criteria

JG's problems certainly interfered with independence in feeding and mobility. Although there may be a cognitive component to the delays, a sensorimotor base to her motor difficulties certainly exists. Previous therapy focused on sitting but did not address mobility. Self-feeding had been

inconsistently attempted by a succession of several therapists in the previous 4 months. Given this, it was decided to
try a period of 3 months of therapy with one consistent occupational therapist focusing on self-feeding and a physical
therapist focusing on mobility.

Treatment Plan

The treatment plan focused on mobility. Mobilization of the tight
joints, followed by reassessment of the muscle flexibility issue
was the first objective. Once the flexibility for standing was available, standing was attempted. Activities focused on eccentric
and concentric strength near the end range for the hip and knee
in standing. These were followed by activities that focused on
gaining concentric and eccentric strength to raise one leg while
supporting on the other. Finally, a walker was introduced.

Results

Movement through the full range of motion was achieved
within the first couple of weeks. By the end of the first month,
JG was able to stand at the couch if her knees were supported. A walker was ordered. By the end of the third month,
JG was able to rise from a small stool to the walker and
ambulate 10 feet while the therapist supported the right hip
as the left leg was brought forward. At this point, it appeared
that an AFO might decrease the effort required of the right leg
to swing the left leg through; the left dorsiflexors still did not
come in fast or frequently enough for JG's preferred speed of
mobility. By the end of the fifth month, JG was able to ambulate 30 feet with the left AFO and walker. However, after two
attempts, she showed an increase in tripping on the right as
she had difficulty clearing the right foot after 40–50 feet of
ambulation. A right AFO was obtained. By 9 months of therapy, JG was able to independently rise from the stool to the
walker and then ambulate from the kitchen to the den and
her bedroom and back (in a reasonable time) using her
walker and AFOs. She still needed someone to keep her focus
on where she was going.

Exit Criteria

In this case example, the mobility goal was achieved. At this point, any adult could help JG practice her ambulation. The bigger concern was how to apply the ambulation in therapy to ambulation as a means of getting around in daily activity. JG was now expected to come to the kitchen from the den for a meal. She also began school. Physical therapy was not needed to teach JG to walk. However, the school provided the environment to make the ambulation functional outside of therapy.

7

Medical Efficiency and Fiscal Responsibility: How to Bill and Be Reimbursed Effectively

Physical and occupational therapists are traditionally trained in assessment and treatment skills; they are trained to a lesser extent in clinical research and documentation skills. The physical and occupational therapy disciplines have been challenged by reimbursement sources to document the medical efficiency and fiscal responsibility of their approaches. These challenges frequently question whether therapy is appropriate (i.e., effective and efficient) and whether alternative resources are more appropriate. They also question the frequency and duration of services. Answers to challenges such as these constitute entrance and exit criteria for services. Entrance and exit criteria are guidelines that insurers, schools, and others use to determine medical efficiency and financial responsibility. Efficient use of resources and logical entrance and exit criteria provide a strong reimbursement strategy to use with insurers, schools, and state Medicaid programs. This chapter explores the concepts of entrance and exit criteria, theoretical and research-based entrance and exit criteria, and frequency and duration criteria, and then applies these concepts to case examples and documentation for reimbursement.

Discussions of guidelines for therapy exist in every state's education department and every insurance company's utilization department. It is not a new topic, yet research that addresses this issue is limited. Research has focused on efficacy of individual therapy styles. Studies regarding the efficacy of certain theoretical perspectives often have limited documentation of whether one approach is better than another (Campbell 1989; Harris et al. 1987; Ottenbacher 1982; Ottenbacher et al. 1986; Ottenbacher and Peterson 1983; Palisano 1991; Palmer et al. 1988; Parette and Hourcade 1984). Other issues, such as when a child benefits, when a child does not benefit, and the frequency and duration necessary to effect a motor performance change, have not been well studied.

Given the limitations of these studies, the question remains: Does exercise, planned with specific goals and techniques, affect motor performance? If so, how much exercise, for how long, and under how much supervision is needed to be effective? Is it necessary for therapy to be supervised by a therapist, or can activities planned in a preschool be equally therapeutic? This chapter discusses issues of the effectiveness of exercise and therapy in general and puts them in the perspective of a decision model for entrance and exit criteria for therapy. The basis of entrance and exit criteria that are applied in the clinical setting is formed from these topics.

Exercise Prescriptions: Guidelines, Frequency, and Duration

Guidelines, frequency, and duration have been addressed in a few sources. Levine and Kliebhan (1981) discussed guidelines for pediatric therapy based on diagnosis, prognosis, and treatment options. Patricia Montgomery (1994) explored the issue of guidelines for frequency and duration of therapy. She raised seven issues that are discussed relative to the case examples in Chapter 6:

1. When a child's progress is slow and much repetition is necessary for learning, should the frequency of direct physical

therapy be reduced? Children with mental retardation learn to move at a rate commensurate with their cognitive abilities. In these cases, therapy has not been shown to enhance the rate of skill acquisition. The case of SI is a classic example of a child whose progress is related to her cognitive abilities, not therapeutic intervention. Therapy was much less beneficial than adapting things in her environment to match her needs (e.g., supplying her with a calculator and telephone with larger buttons).

2.   How many months or years should we continue to provide physical therapy that is primarily passive (maximum handling) when children continue to show limited motivation or ability for self-initiated movement? Therapy that coordinates with the interest and willingness of the child may be more beneficial than repetitive therapy that takes place when the child is uninterested or unwilling to participate. Limited motivation certainly affected the speed at which CA gained independence in his environment; inability to initiate most mobility limited RS's independence. Changing CA's motivation to move was relatively easy when his environment, age, and interests were taken into account. CA was much more willing to walk to his friend's house than around the gym (an equivalent distance). The nature of RS's disorder prevents him from improving his motor skills substantially. That does not mean therapy is unwarranted but perhaps should be redirected and decreased. Instead of focusing on twice-weekly therapy to teach this 3-year-old gifted child to roll (a skill he cannot accomplish), perhaps a consultative therapy model that focuses on adapting his computer, so he can turn it on and off independently, would be more useful.

3.   Should we continue to provide physical therapy to children in environments that may diminish the effectiveness of our interventions? Therapy provided in settings where children play provides the "tools" the children continue to use when not in therapy. Hence, services provided in hospitals with therapy equipment (as JB and CA initially received)—or in isolated classrooms away from

the toys and architectural barriers they frequently encounter—may not be as effective as services provided in more natural settings. JB and CA benefited from the replacement of less frequent, structured therapy with more age-appropriate and socially appropriate activities involving participation in preschool and community activities.

4. Are we expecting too much—or too little—of caregivers? Each child has a unique set of social supports, whether it be a single parent, extended family, church, and community support. Frequency of therapy may be appropriately adjusted based not only on the child's direct response to the therapist but also on the child's response to his or her own environmental supports.

5. Is high-frequency, direct physical therapy that occurs over long periods generally unwarranted and cost-ineffective for progressive and genetic disorders? The natural history of many disorders has been clearly documented. Direct extensive therapy over long periods has not been shown to influence the outcome of Werdnig-Hoffmann's disease (spinal muscular atrophy type I), muscular dystrophy, Down syndrome, and many other progressive or genetic disorders. Although specific individuals may show more response to intervention than others, a consultative model may be more effective in terms of the child's time and quality of life and the family's financial resources.

6. How effectively do we use a child's age as a guide for physical therapy intervention? There is little argument that focusing therapeutic intervention in the first 3 years is beneficial from an educational perspective (Bloom 1964), a normal developmental perspective (Bailey 1993; Gesell 1947; McGraw 1945; Ramey et al. 1987), a treatment perspective (Ayres 1972; Bobath 1980; Rood in Stockmeyer 1967), and a physiologic perspective. It is the rigid adherence to a developmental sequence of a child regardless of his or her age that has come into question. Molnar (1988) suggests guidelines to adjust the focus of therapy to the child's chronologic age. Younger children, thought to have more neural plasticity, may benefit from therapy focused on facilitating "normal" movement.

However, if "normal" movement has not progressed for the older child, alternative methods are necessary to allow the child to interact with the environment and to minimize environmental retardation and trained social dependence.

7. Should the therapist help the child achieve motor skills at the highest level of independence possible, without specifying how? "As children with developmental disabilities age, a history of the frequency and duration of intervention in relation to rate of progress can be documented. This history provides data on which to base future recommendations" (Montgomery 1994, p. 47). Future recommendations must be geared toward providing functional independence for the child within the bounds of the natural history of the disorder. Montgomery cites a classic example:

> *For example, the physical therapist's goal may be for the child with spastic diplegia to walk with a more neutral pelvis and a better heel-strike (e.g., decreased anterior pelvic tilt and decreased toe-walking); however, the child's goal may be to walk independently from point A to point B as quickly as possible to keep up with peers. In this case, several questions arise: 1. Can the gait pattern desired by the physical therapist be achieved at all? In other words, what is the natural history of the developing gait pattern in cerebral palsy, and how much can it be altered, even with the most intensive interventions? 2. How much physical therapy will be required to achieve the therapist's goal (e.g., weekly frequency with a duration of months or years)? Is this a cost-effective goal? 3. Is the goal meaningful to the child or the family? 4. Will this improved gait, if achieved, be functional? Will the child be able to use the gait pattern naturally, or will it require excessive concentration and increased energy expenditure? (p. 47)*

HS's case provides a similar example. His rate of change is consistent over time in fine and gross motor, speech, and adaptive skills. He scored consistently at 50% of norms in all domains every year he was tested. His gain in skills appears to be developmental and not related to therapy; did he benefit from the therapy? Did the therapy take away from other, perhaps more useful, activities? Although maximizing function without focusing on how the function is achieved may be controversial to therapists, it is not controversial to funding sources or to the child.

Courts have even become involved as parents sue school districts over service issues. In response to this, many state education departments have developed entrance and exit guidelines, but few have developed specific criteria.

Criteria

In a major local conference, some competing therapy groups were trying to convince seven large insurers in the area to develop a contract with them; the medical director of one of the insurers explained that there was no need to develop a contract with them because the agency the seven currently had a contract with was "medically efficient and fiscally responsible." The insurers were willing to pay for services that were medically necessary, responsive to therapy, and required the special skills of a therapist. This is medical efficiency. Fiscal responsibility of the agency, over the child's lifespan, is to provide services when the child is benefiting and reduce services at times when the child is not benefiting by allowing the child to enter and exit services as needed and by coordinating therapy with therapeutic lifestyles.

Medical efficiency occurs when relevant medical (or educational, depending on your perspective and employer) services are provided to children (with a diagnosis), and the response to those services demonstrates improvement related to the service—a service that cannot be provided through other means. This is the basis for entrance criteria for medical- or school-based therapy.

The criteria used in this text were developed by the Iowa Department of Education in response to a suit filed by parents concerned with frequency and duration of therapy. The department put together a panel made up of four therapists, one from outside the state, two in the state working for local education areas (LEAs) other than the one involved, and one from the LEA involved. Two administrators, two parents, and many state therapists were available for input. The panel developed criteria based on 20 cases, including the 13 involved in the lawsuit. The therapist panel assessed each child individually; each therapist independently determined his or her own recommendations; then the panel discussed the rationale for their recommendations in terms of the child's response to therapy and the diagnosis, prognosis, and relevance of the therapy. Their criteria were then field tested by school therapists across Iowa. The recommendations from the field testers were addressed in the final phase of the criteria development. These criteria were related to the case examples presented in Chapter 6. Several of these criteria are explored here.

1.   Medical or educational relevance: Therapy must relate to something in the child's life and be consistent with the development of motor control that was presented in Chapter 3. The therapist must clearly identify the goal relative to the child. Range of motion and strengthening are not the child's goals. The knowledge of the ability to move from classroom to lunchroom with peers is a pertinent *educational*, not medical, goal. Proper ambulation is the *medical* goal for a child who does not ambulate functionally at school.

2.   Relevance of therapy in light of diagnosis and prognosis: Continued therapy against physiologically impossible odds does nothing for the child and may in fact be physically and emotionally harmful.

3.   Response to therapy and length of time for response: Is more therapy over a longer time necessary or better than either concentrated therapy with breaks or a consultative model of therapy? One must consider how much time elapses before change occurs and whether that change may be related to other factors

such as cognitive development (as in HS's case). Might there be a point at which changes in the child's environment should be attempted (e.g., adaptive equipment or modifications made for SI)? When limited success is found following a given treatment regimen, alternative approaches may be more productive, as in the examples of HS, SI, and JG.

4. Improvement relates to therapy, not other factors: Improvement may also be related to other factors such as maturity, cognitive development, or behavior management. Compare the examples of SI and HS with JG and NY: SI and HS had issues with cognitive development and behavior (respectively), not with range, strength, or motor planning. JG and NY quickly showed marked improvement in their motor performance when the therapeutic activities changed. Improvement appeared to be related to therapy for JG and NY but not for SI and HS.

5. Therapy versus therapeutic lifestyle: Does the child need the special skills of the therapist or can the same skills be gained in the child's natural environment? At what point should one be substituted for the other? Once CA was walking, endurance could be attained in his lifestyle activities (e.g., walking to his friend's house). In contrast, JB could build endurance in his lifestyle activities but still required monthly to quarterly intervention from therapy; his periods of relatively greater immobility and rapid growth resulted in musculoskeletal changes that he could not overcome alone.

Frequency can be determined from examination. Frequency determined partly from consultation with family, teachers, or other therapists can suggest either an interdisciplinary or transdisciplinary model of therapy. Patterns of frequency may be steady over time or concentrated, perhaps with breaks between concentrated sessions. Given the limited research on general efficacy, it is not surprising that there has been even less research on frequency or patterns of frequency. Clinical documentation and creativity are still needed to develop a guide for decision making in this area.

Exit Criteria

A concept given little attention in the literature is exit criteria. Decisions to begin therapy are often clear, but criteria for ending therapy are often subjective or based more on hope than reality. More objective exit criteria are a natural extension of entrance criteria. Exit criteria do not pertain to an end point but rather a pause point for many children because, as children grow, their needs change, often qualifying them for additional therapy. Exit criteria identified by the Iowa panel include completion of child's goals, potential for further change, cessation of the problem as an issue in the child's life, or contraindication of therapy owing to a change in medical or educational status.

The first exit criterion is completion of the child's goals. Goals must be appropriate for the age and cognition of the child; they should also be appropriate to the family input. Heel-toe gait in an 18-month-old is inappropriate, as heel-strike is not normal at that age. In the case examples, CA had reached his goal. New goals were not appropriate at that time.

The second criterion is potential for further change. RS's potential for further change through therapy is limited, but change through technology may still be possible. Rather than continued therapy, referral to a teacher or an adaptive technology specialist may be appropriate. RS's limitation is clear because it is related to the prognosis for his disorder. Determining the potential for change in a child such as NY is not as easy. Little potential exists for gaining strength in NY's gastrocnemius soleus. She has worked toward this goal for 3 years and made little progress. Because there was only a trace response to tickle in the gastrocnemius soleus group, it is unlikely she will be able to gain enough strength in the muscle for use in a functional gait. In her case, the use of the AFOs is more efficient and effective than twice-weekly therapy (in hope of achieving ambulation without the AFOs).

The third criterion is that the problem ceases to be an issue in the child's life. Working on crawling when the 30-month-old child is trying to stand and cruise (JG), working on ambulation when an electric wheelchair is purchased, practicing handwriting when the child is in high school or has limited motor ability to write and uses a computer such as RS, are all examples of times when this exit criterion may apply.

The final criterion is that the therapy becomes contraindicated due to a change in medical or educational status. For example, the therapeutic program as designed may become irrelevant or inappropriate when the child moves to a different classroom with different goals.

Bibliography

Ayres A. Sensory Integration and Learning Disorders. Los Angeles: Western Psychological Services, 1972.

Bailey N. Bailey Scales of Infant Development (2nd ed). San Antonio, TX: The Psychological Corporation, 1993.

Bernstein N. Coordination and Regulation of Movements. New York: Pergamon, 1967.

Bleck E. Developmental orthopaedics. III: toddlers. Dev Med Child Neurol 1982;24:533–555.

Bloom R. Stability and Change in Human Characteristics. New York: John Wiley & Sons, 1964.

Bobath K. A Neurophysiological Basis for the Treatment of Cerebral Palsy. Philadelphia: Lippincott, 1980.

Bottos M, Dalla B, Stefani D, et al. Locomotor strategies preceding independent walking: prospective study of neurological and language development in 424 cases. Dev Med Child Neurol 1989;31:25–34.

Bradley N, Bekoff A. Development of Locomotion: Animal Models. In M Wollacott, A Shumway-Cook (eds), The Development of Posture and Gait across the Life Span. Columbia, SC: University of South Carolina Press, 1989.

Brooks S. Hip joint limitation: contribution to sacral sitting. Dev Med Child Neurol 1990;43:84. Poster presented at the national conference of the American Academy of Cerebral Palsy and Developmental Medicine, June 1990.

Brooks S. Suggestions from the field: hip joint limitation: contribution to sacral sitting. Pediatr Phys Ther 1994;6:92.

Brooks-Scott S. Joint Mobilization for the Neurologically Involved Child [videotape]. Albuquerque, NM: Clinician's View, 1998.

Brooks-Scott S. Joint Mobilization in the Child with Neurological Impairment [videotape]. Albuquerque, NM: Clinician's View, 1998.

Campbell S. [Editorial]. Phys Occup Ther Pediatr 1989;9:1–4.

Cavanaugh P, Kram R. The efficiency of human movement—a statement of the problem. Med Sci Sports Exerc 1985;17:304–308.

Cornwall M. Biomechanics of noncontractile tissue. A review. Phys Ther 1984;63:1869–1873.

Craik R. Abnormalities of Motor Behavior in Contemporary Management of Motor Control Problems: Proceedings of the II Step Conference. Alexandria, VA: Foundation for Physical Therapy, 1991;155–164.

Cusick B. Progressive Casting and Splinting for Lower Extremity Deformities in Children with Neuromotor Dysfunction. The Denver Developmental Scales Test. Tucson, AZ: Skillbuild, 1990.

Dietz V, Ketelsen U, Berger W, Quintern E. Motor unit involvement in spastic paresis: relationship between leg muscle activation and histochemistry. J Neurol Sci 1986;75:89–103.

Edström L, Grimby L, Hannerz J. Correlation between recruitment order of motor units and muscle atrophy pattern in upper motoneuron lesion: significance of spasticity. Experimentia 1973; 29:560–561.

Frankenburg W, Dodds J. The Denver Developmental Scales Test. J Pediatr 1967;71:181.

Gate V, Stefanova-Uzunova M, Stamatova L, Ivonov I. Excitation-contraction latency in the muscles of children and adults. Dev Med Child Neurol 1986;28:642–645.

Gesell A, Amatruda C. Developmental Diagnosis. New York: Hoeber, 1947.

Guiliani C. Theories of Motor Control: New Concepts for Physical Therapy in Contemporary Management of Motor Control Problems: Proceedings of the II Step Conference. Alexandria, VA: Foundation for Physical Therapy, 1991;29–36.

Haas S, Epps C, Adams J. Normal ranges of hip motion in the newborn. Clin Orthop Relat Res 1973;91:114–118.

Harris S, Atwater S, Crowe T. Accepted and controversial neuromotor therapies for infants at high-risk for cerebral palsy. J Perinatol 1987;8:3–13.

Harris S, Lundgren B. Joint mobilization for children with central nervous system disorders: indications and precautions. Phys Ther 1991;71:890–896.

Hensinger R, Jone E. Developmental orthopedics I: the lower limb. Dev Med Child Neurol 1982;24:95–116.

Heriza C. Motor Development: Traditional and Contemporary Theories in Contemporary Management of Motor Control Problems: Proceedings of the II Step Conference. Alexandria, VA: Foundation for Physical Therapy, 1991;99–126.

Hoesli B. Effects of mobilization on hip flexion range in a child with cerebral palsy. Paper presented at the American Physical Therapy Association National Conference, June 1989.

Hoffer M. Joint motion limitation in newborns. Clin Orthop Rel Res 1980;148:94–96.

Horak F. Assumptions Underlying Motor Control for Neurologic Rehabilitation in Contemporary Management of Motor Control

Problems: Proceedings of the II Step Conference. Alexandria, VA: Foundation for Physical Therapy, 1991;11–28.

Hoy M, Zernicke R. The role of intersegmental dynamics during rapid limb oscillations. J Biomech 1986;19:867–877.

Hoy M, Zernicke R, Smith J. Contrasting roles of inertial and muscular moments at ankle and knee during paw-shake response. J Neurophysiol 1985;54:1282–1294.

Jackson J, Taylor J (eds). Selected Writings of John B. Hughlings, I and II. London: Hodder & Stoughter, 1932.

Keshner E. How Theoretical Framework Biases Evaluation and Treatment in Contemporary Management of Motor Control Problems: Proceedings of the II Step Conference. Alexandria, VA: Foundation for Physical Therapy, 1991;37–48.

Kessler R, Hertling D. Management of Common Musculoskeletal Disorders. Philadelphia: Harper & Row, 1983.

Kramer J, MacPhail A. Relationships among measures of walking efficiency, gross motor ability, and isokinetic strength in adolescents with cerebral palsy. Pediatr Phys Ther 1994;6:3–9.

Lee C. Forces acting to derotate exaggerated femoral anteversion in the newborn hip [thesis of fellowship]. Stanford, NY: UCP Research, Ed. Foundation NY Children's Hospital, 1977.

LeVeau B, Bernhardt D. Developmental biomechanics: effect of forces on the growth, development, and maintenance of the human body. Phys Ther 1984;64:1874–1882.

Levine MS, Kliebhan L. Communication between physician and physical and occupational therapists: a neurodevelopmentally based prescription. Pediatrics 1981;68:208–214.

Lockman J, Thelen E. Developmental biodynamics: brain, body, behavior connections. Child Dev 1993;64:953–959.

Maitland G. Peripheral Manipulation (vol 2). Boston: Butterworth, 1977.

Malina R. Racial/ethnic variation in the motor development and performances of American children. Can J Sport Sci 1998;13(2):136–143.

McCrea J. Pediatric Orthopedics of the Lower Extremity: An Instructional Handbook. Mount Kisco, NY: Futura Publishing, 1985.

McGraw M. Neuromuscular Maturation of the Human Infant. New York: Hafner Publishing, 1945.

Molnar G. A developmental perspective for the rehabilitation of children with physical disability. Pediatr Ann 1988;17:766–776.

Montgomery P. Helping families obtain physical therapy for their children with developmental disabilities while also helping to contain costs: a clinician asks some hard questions. PT Mag 1994;(March 19):42–47, 89–91.

Nelson W. Physical principles for economies of skilled movements. Biol Cybern 1983;46:135–147.

Ottenbacher K. Sensory integration therapy: affect or effect. Am J Occup Ther 1982;36:571–578.

Ottenbacher K, Biocca Z, DeCremer G, et al. Quantitative analysis of the effectiveness of pediatric therapy: emphasis on neurodevelopmental treatment approach. Phys Ther 1986;66:1095–1101.

Ottenbacher K, Peterson P. The efficacy of vestibular stimulation as a form of specific sensory enrichment. Clin Pediatr (Phila) 1983;23:428–433.

Palisano R. Research on the effectiveness of neurodevelopmental treatment. Pediatr Phys Ther 1991;3:1443–1448.

Palmer F, Shapiro B, Wachtel R, et al. The effects of physical therapy on cerebral palsy: a controlled trial in infants with spastic diplegia. N Engl J Med 1988;318:803–808.

Parette H, Hourcade J. A review of therapeutic intervention research on gross and fine motor progress in young children with cerebral palsy. Am J Occup Ther 1984;38:462–468.

Pearson P, Williams C. Physical Therapy Services in the Developmental Disabilities. Springfield, IL: Thomas, 1972.

Piaget J, Inhelder B. The Gaps in Empiricism. In A Kostler, J Smythies (eds), Beyond Reductionism: New Perspectives in the Life Sciences. New York: MacMillan, 1969;118–148.

Polit A, Bizzi E. Characteristics of motor programs underlying arm movements in monkeys. J Neurophysiol 1979;42:183–194.

Ramey C, Best D, Suarez T. Early Intervention: Why, for Whom, How, at What Cost? In N Gunzenhauser (ed), Infant Stimulation: For Whom, What Kind, When and How Much? Pediatric Round Table 13. Skillman, NJ: Johnson & Johnson Baby Products, 1987;170–180.

Robson P. Prewalking locomotor movements and their use in predicting standing and walking. Child Care Health Dev 1984;10: 317–330.

Schmidt R. Motor Learning Principles for Physical Therapy in Contemporary Management of Motor Control Problems: Proceedings of the II Step Conference. Alexandria, VA: Foundation for Physical Therapy, 1991;49–64.

Schneider K, Zernicke R. A FORTRAN package for the planar analysis of limb intersegmental dynamics from spatial coordinate-time data. Adv Eng Software 1990;12:1123–1128.

Schneider K, Zernicke R, Ulrich B, et al. Understanding movement control in infants through the analysis of limb intersegmental dynamics. J Mot Behav 1990;22:493–520.

Sgarlato T. A Compendium of Biomechanics. San Francisco: College of Podiatric Medicine, 1971.

Sherrington C. The Integrative Action of the Nervous System. New Haven, CT: Yale University Press, 1906.

Smith J, Zernicke R. Predictions for neural control based on limb dynamics. Trends Neurosci 1987;10:123–128.

Spaans F, Wilts G. Denervation due to lesions of the central nervous system. J Neurol Sci 1982;57:291–305.

Sporns O, Edelman G. Solving Bernstein's problem: a proposal for the development of coordinated movement by selection. Child Dev 1993;64:960–981.

Stockmeyer S. An interpretation of the approach of Rood to the treatment of neuromuscular dysfunction. Am J Phys Med 1967;46:901–956.

Super C. Environmental effects on moor development: the case of "African infant precocity." Dev Med Child Neurol 1976;18: 561–567.

Tardieu G, Tardieu C. Cerebral palsy: mechanical evaluation and conservative correction of limb joint contractures. Clin Orthop Rel Res 1987;219:63–70.

Thelen E, Corbetta D, Kamm K, et al. The transition of reaching: mapping intention and intrinsic dynamics. Child Dev 1993;64:1058–1098.

Thorton K. Screening Moroccan infants using the Wolanski Gross Motor Evaluation: a pilot study. Stud Hum Ecol 1992;10:121–126.

Threlkeld A. The effects of manual therapy on connective tissue. Phys Ther 1992;72:893–902.

Towen C. Primitive reflexes—conceptual or semantic problem? Clin Dev Med 1984;94:115–125.

Tuller B, Turvey M, Fitch H. The Bernstein Perspective II: The Concept of Muscle Linkage or Coordinative Structure. In J Kelso (ed), Human Motor Behavior: An Introduction. Hillsdale, NJ: Lawrence Erlbaum Associates, 1982;239–252.

Turvey M, Fitch H, Tuller B. The Bernstein Perspective in Human Behavior. In J Kelso (ed), Human Motor Behavior: An Introduction. Hillsdale, NJ: Lawrence Erlbaum Associates, 1982;239–252.

Vaughn V. Effects of upper limb immobilization on isometric strength, movement time, and triphasic electromyographic characteristics. Phys Ther 1989;69(2):119–129.

Voss D, Ionta M, Myers B. Proprioceptive Neuromuscular Facilitation: Patterns and Techniques (3rd ed). Philadelphia: Lippincott-Raven, 1985.

Zernicke R, Schneider K. Biomechanics and developmental neuromotor control. Child Dev 1993;64:982–1004.

Index

Assessment
  clinical protocols for, 47–54
  dynamic systems approach (Heriza), 47–48
  normal range of motion values for children, 50–51, 52
  proposed functional strength criteria for children, 53
  sacral sitting vs. normal sitting, 49–50, 51
Ayres, and theory of sensory integration, 5

Bernstein, and interactions between musculoskeletal and nervous systems, 8, 9, 13
Billing and reimbursement, 79–88
  criteria for, 84–87
    improvement relates to therapy and not other factors, 86
    medical or educational relevance, 85
    relevance of therapy in light of diagnosis and prognosis, 85
    response to therapy and length of time for response, 85–86
    therapy vs. therapeutic lifestyle, 86
  exercise prescriptions, 80–84
  exit criteria for, 87–88
    completion of child's goals, 87
    potential for further change, 87–88
    problem ceases to be issue for child, 88
    therapy becomes contraindicated due to change in medical or educational status, 88
  limitations of research and, 79–80
  medical efficiency and, 84
Biomechanics of motor control, 13–20
  basic principles of, 14–18
    control of reach
      in adults, 18–19
      in infants, 19–20
    muscle, viscoelastic properties of, 16–18
    passive components of musculoskeletal system, 14–15
Bobath, and neurodevelopmental treatment approach, 1. *See also*
        Neurodevelopmental treatment approach
Bone
  biomechanics and, 14–15
  growth of, in child with neurologic insult, 22

Brooks, and improvements in sitting, 44

Cartilage, biomechanics and, 15
Cerebral palsy, classic history of, 21
Closed-pack, open-pack positions, 26
Collagenous tissues, biomechanics and, 15
Contractures, appropriate techniques for, 28
Criteria for therapy. *See* Billing and reimbursement, criteria for

Dynamic systems theory, 8–9
Dynamics, 14

Efficiency of movement, 18
Exercise prescriptions, 80–84
Exit criteria, 87–88

Feedback and feed-forward systems, 7–8
Force, 16

Grades of motion, 25–26
Guiliani, and dynamic systems theory, 8–9.

Heriza, and assessment of children with motor dysfunction, 47–48
Hip joint, 23
Hoesli, inferior glide and effect on sitting, 44
Horak, and assumptions about motor control, 5

Iowa Department of Education criteria. *See* Billing and reimbursement,
       criteria for

Joint formation, in children with neurologic insult, 22–23
Joint play, 25

Kinematics, 14

Mobilization
    choosing appropriate technique of, 28
    effectiveness of, 44–45
    indications and contraindications, 26–28
    principles of, 24–43. *See also* Orthopedic assessment
        closed-pack, open-pack positions, 26
        grades of motion, 25–26